Renal Complications in the Catheterization Laboratory

Editors

HITINDER S. GURM
JUDITH KOOIMAN

INTERVENTIONAL CARDIOLOGY CLINICS

www.interventional.theclinics.com

Consulting Editors
SAMIN K. SHARMA
IGOR F. PALACIOS

July 2014 • Volume 3 • Number 3

ELSEVIER

1600 John F. Kennedy Boulevard • Suite 1800 • Philadelphia, Pennsylvania, 19103-2899

http://www.theclinics.com

INTERVENTIONAL CARDIOLOGY CLINICS Volume 3, Number 3
July 2014 ISSN 2211-7458, ISBN-13: 978-0-323-31329-2

Editor: Adrianne Brigido
Developmental Editor: Barbara Cohen-Kligerman

Interventional Cardiology Clinics (ISSN 2211-7458) is published quarterly by Elsevier Inc., 360 Park Avenue South, New York, NY 10010-1710. Months of issue are January, April, July, and October. Subscription prices are USD 195 per year for US individuals, USD 305 for US institutions, USD 130 per year for US students, USD 230 per year for Canadian individuals, USD 375 for Canadian institutions, USD 150 per year for Canadian students, USD 295 per year for international individuals, USD 375 for international institutions, and USD 150 per year for international students. To receive student/resident rate, orders must be accompanied by name of affiliated institution, date of term, and the *signature* of program/residency coordinator on institution letterhead. Orders will be billed at individual rate until proof of status is received. Foreign air speed delivery is included in all *Clinics* subscription prices. All prices are subject to change without notice. **POSTMASTER:** Send address changes to *Interventional Cardiology Clinics*, Elsevier Health Sciences Division, Subscription Customer Service, 3251 Riverport Lane, Maryland Heights, MO 63043. **Customer Service: Telephone: 1-800-654-2452** (U.S. and Canada); **1-314-447-8871** (outside U.S. and Canada). **Fax: 1-314-447-8029. E-mail: journalscustomerservice-usa@elsevier.com** (for print support); **journalsonlinesupport-usa@elsevier.com** (for online support).

Reprints. For copies of 100 or more of articles in this publication, please contact the Commercial Reprints Department, Elsevier Inc., 360 Park Avenue South, New York, NY 10010-1710. Tel.: 212-633-3874; Fax: 212-633-3820; E-mail: reprints@elsevier.com.

Contributors

CONSULTING EDITORS

SAMIN K. SHARMA, MD, FSCAI, FACC
Director of Clinical Cardiology; Director of
Cardiac Catheterization Laboratory, Mount
Sinai Medical Center, New York, New York

IGOR F. PALACIOS, MD, FSCAI
Director of Interventional Cardiology,
Cardiology Division, Heart Center,
Massachusetts General Hospital; Associate
Professor of Medicine, Harvard Medical
School, Boston, Massachusetts

EDITORS

HITINDER S. GURM, MD
University of Michigan Cardiovascular Center,
Division of Cardiovascular Medicine,
Department of Internal Medicine, Frankel
Cardiovascular Center, University of Michigan
Health System, Ann Arbor, Michigan

JUDITH KOOIMAN, MSc
Department of Thrombosis and Hemostasis;
Department of Nephrology, Leiden University
Medical Center, Leiden, South Holland,
The Netherlands

AUTHORS

IRAM AQEEL, MD
Renal, Electrolyte and Hypertension Division,
University of Pennsylvania, Philadelphia,
Pennsylvania

PETER ASPELIN, MD, PhD
Professor, Division of Medical Imaging and
Technology, Department of Clinical Science,
Intervention and Technology, Karolinska
University Hospital, Karolinska Institutet,
Stockholm, Sweden

**HANNA BACHORZEWSKA-GAJEWSKA,
MD, PhD**
Professor, Department of Invasive Cardiology,
Medical University, Bialystok, Poland

ROBERT M. BELL, BSc, PhD, MRCP
General and Interventional Cardiology
Department, The Heart Hospital, University
College Hospitals NHS Trust; NIHR Academic
Lecturer, Clinical Research Department, The
Hatter Cardiovascular Institute, University
College London, London, United Kingdom

FRANCESCO BELLANDI, MD
Cardiology Division, Prato Hospital, Prato, Italy

MICHAEL BUSCHUR, MD
Interventional Cardiology Fellow, Division of
Cardiovascular Medicine, University of
Michigan, Ann Arbor, Michigan

SLAWOMIR DOBRZYCKI, MD, PhD
Professor, Department of Invasive Cardiology,
Medical University, Bialystok, Poland

STEPHEN J. DUFFY, MBBS, PhD
Cardiovascular Medicine, Baker IDI Heart and
Diabetes Institute, Alfred Hospital, Melbourne,
Victoria, Australia

JUSTIN M. DUNN, MD, MPH
Interventional Cardiology Fellow, Cleveland
Clinic, Cleveland, Ohio

AMARINDER S. GARCHA, MD
Renal, Electrolyte and Hypertension Division,
University of Pennsylvania, Philadelphia,
Pennsylvania

REMY W.F. GEENEN, MD
Department of Radiology, Medisch Centrum Alkmaar, Alkmaar, Netherlands

SACHIN S. GOEL, MD
Interventional Cardiology, Department of Cardiovascular Medicine, Heart & Vascular Institute, Cleveland, Ohio

HITINDER S. GURM, MD
University of Michigan Cardiovascular Center, Division of Cardiovascular Medicine, Department of Internal Medicine, Frankel Cardiovascular Center, University of Michigan Health System, Ann Arbor, Michigan

MICHAEL HOWE, MD
Cardiovascular Medicine Fellow, Division of Cardiovascular Medicine, Department of Internal Medicine, Frankel Cardiovascular Center, University of Michigan Health System, Ann Arbor, Michigan

SAMIR R. KAPADIA, MD
Professor of Medicine; Director, Cardiac Catheterization Laboratory, Cleveland Clinic, Cleveland, Ohio

DAVID M. KAYE, MBBS, PhD, FACC
Cardiovascular Medicine, Baker IDI Heart and Diabetes Institute, Alfred Hospital, Melbourne, Victoria, Australia

HYLKE JAN KINGMA, PharmD
Department of Clinical Pharmacy, Stichting Apotheek der Haarlemse Ziekenhuizen, Haarlem, Netherlands

JUDITH KOOIMAN, MSc
Department of Thrombosis and Hemostasis; Department of Nephrology, Leiden University Medical Center, Leiden, South Holland, The Netherlands

MARIO LEONCINI, MD
Cardiology Division, Prato Hospital, Prato, Italy

MAURO MAIOLI, MD
Cardiology Division, Prato Hospital, Prato, Italy

JOLANTA MALYSZKO, MD, PhD
Professor, Second Department of Nephrology, Medical University, Bialystok, Poland

DAMIEN MARYCZ, MD
Division of Cardiovascular Medicine, Gill Heart Institute, University of Kentucky, Lexington, Kentucky

PETER A. MCCULLOUGH, MD, MPH, FACC, FACP, FAHA, FCCP, FNKF
Baylor University Medical Center, Baylor Heart and Vascular Institute, Baylor Jack and Jane Hamilton Heart and Vascular Hospital, Dallas, Texas; The Heart Hospital, Plano, Texas

PASCAL MEIER, MD
Assistant Professor Adjunct in Cardiovascular Medicine, Yale School of Medicine; General and Interventional Cardiology Department, The Heart Hospital, University College Hospitals NHS Trust, London, United Kingdom

ROGER REAR, BSc, MRCP
General and Interventional Cardiology Department, The Heart Hospital, University College Hospitals NHS Trust; Clinical Research Associate, Clinical Research Department, The Hatter Cardiovascular Institute, University College London, London, United Kingdom

IGOR ROJKOVSKIY, MD
Division of Nephrology and Hypertension, Fletcher Allen Health Care, University of Vermont College of Medicine, Burlington, Vermont

MICHAEL R. RUDNICK, MD, FACP
Renal, Electrolyte and Hypertension Division, University of Pennsylvania, Philadelphia, Pennsylvania

MEHDI H. SHISHEHBOR, DO, MPH, PhD
Director, Endovascular Services, Heart & Vascular Institute, Cleveland Clinic, Cleveland, Ohio

RICHARD SOLOMON, MD, FASN, FACP
Director, Division of Nephrology and Hypertension, Fletcher Allen Health Care; Patrick Professor of Medicine, University of Vermont College of Medicine, Burlington, Vermont

DION STUB, MBBS, PhD
Cardiovascular Medicine, Baker IDI Heart and Diabetes Institute, Alfred Hospital, Melbourne, Victoria, Australia

ANNA TOSO, MD
Cardiology Division, Prato Hospital, Prato, Italy

FRANCESCO TROPEANO, MD
Cardiology Division, Prato Hospital, Prato, Italy

E. MURAT TUZCU, MD
Professor of Medicine; Vice Chairman of Cardiovascular Medicine, Cleveland Clinic, Cleveland, Ohio

AART J. VAN DER MOLEN, MD
Department of Radiology, Leiden University Medical Center, Leiden, Netherlands

KHALED M. ZIADA, MD
Division of Cardiovascular Medicine, Gill Heart Institute, University of Kentucky, Lexington, Kentucky

Contents

Traditional cardiovascular risk factors, particularly hypertension and diabetes, are common in the disease processes of both renal and cardiac pathology. Unfortunately the coexistence of renal impairment is not an innocent bystander in cardiovascular disease; this disorder not only increases the prevalence and severity of cardiovascular disease, but also negatively affects prognostic outcomes and the safety and efficacy of cardiac interventions. This article discusses the role and impact of kidney disease in the cardiac patient in 3 key common cardiovascular processes: coronary artery disease, arrhythmia, and heart failure.

Contrast media are essential for cardiac catheterization, and the evolution of these agents has had a significant role in cardiology. Contrast agents are classified as ionic or nonionic based on water solubility and as monomers or dimers based on their chemical structures. Furthermore, these agents are classified on osmolality as high osmolar, low osmolar, or iso-osmolar. The last century has seen a rapid evolution of these agents from their discovery during the search for syphilis treatments to advancements in their chemical properties, making them safer for patients and improving tissue visualization.

Nonrenal complications of contrast media are caused by chemotoxic or anaphylactoid reactions related to the contrast agent used. Chemotoxicity is mainly attributed to ionic concentration and osmolality. Anaphylactoid reactions are typically caused by direct activation of basophils, mast cells, and complement rather than an observable antigen-antibody interaction, and may be acute or delayed. History of an adverse reaction following prior exposure is the strongest predictor of a subsequent adverse reaction to contrast. Premedication regimens of corticosteroids or antihistamines can lower the risk of repeat adverse reactions. Treatment of anaphylactoid reactions depends on the severity of symptoms.

Contrast-induced nephropathy (CIN) is a common cause of acute kidney injury among hospitalized patients. High-osmolar contrast agents are associated with increased risk of CIN. Low-osmolar (LOCM) agents, other than iohexol and ioxaglate, and iso-osmolar (IOCM) agents show no difference in the incidence of CIN, even among high-risk patients. This finding suggests that factors other than osmolality may play a role in the pathogenesis of CIN. The use of either LOCM, with the exception of iohexol and ioxaglate, or IOCM is recommended in high-risk patients.

Contrast-induced nephropathy, now termed contrast-induced acute kidney injury (CI-AKI), has been a long-recognized complication of administering intravascular iodinated contrast. This article reviews the newest literature on subclinical CI-AKI detected by novel biomarkers and clinical CI-AKI recognized by an increase in serum creatinine and a reduction in urine output. Both components of CI-AKI are associated with adverse outcomes, including in-hospital complications, increased length of stay, need for renal replacement therapy, rehospitalization, permanent loss in renal filtration function, and death.

Contrast-induced acute kidney injury (CI-AKI) refers to acute kidney injury (AKI) after intravenous or intra-arterial administration of contrast media (CM). The 2 key mechanisms related to AKI are acute tubular necrosis and prerenal azotemia. Although the pathophysiology of AKI is complex, modern frameworks show that AKI has 3 major pathways: hemodynamic injury, systemic inflammation, and toxic injury. In the pathophysiology of CI-AKI, 3 major distinct, but potentially interacting, pathways are recognized: hemodynamic effects, increase in oxygen free radicals, and direct CM molecule tubular cell toxicity. This article reviews the pathophysiology of CI-AKI by describing and explaining these pathways.

Risk scores should undergo 3 analytical phases before they are suitable for adoption in clinical practice, namely, derivation, external validation, and assessment of effect on clinical outcomes of using the risk score in a so-called impact study. Major risk factors for renal complications after percutaneous coronary intervention are pre-existing chronic kidney disease, diabetes mellitus, use of a high contrast dose, and hemodynamic instability. Unfortunately, only 3 of 10 risk scores have undergone external validation. As a result, there is a great need for further research on the already designed risk scores.

Contrast-induced nephropathy, or contrast-induced acute kidney injury (AKI), is an acute impairment of renal function as manifested by an increase in serum creatinine. Different urinary and serum proteins have been intensively investigated as possible biomarkers for the early diagnosis of AKI. Promising candidate biomarkers have the ability to detect an early and graded increase in tubular epithelial cell injury and to distinguish prerenal causes of AKI from acute tubular necrosis. In this article new, emerging biomarkers of contrast-induced AKI are presented and described. Of these, serum neutrophil gelatinase-associated lipocalin appears to be the most promising.

Prevention of contrast-induced nephropathy is founded on minimizing the pathophysiologic consequences of contrast media (CM) interacting with a vulnerable kidney. In this article, the rationale for administering fluid (oral or intravenous) is discussed, and the clinical trials exploring different protocols are reviewed. A benefit from administration of fluids before CM exposure, which corrects volume depletion and increases urine output, can be expected. Forced diuresis without adequate volume replacement is deleterious.

In the effort to prevent contrast-induced acute kidney injury (CI-AKI), several pharmacologic agents have been tested for their single or combined nephroprotective properties. To date, however, no drug has been officially approved for this aim. This article focuses on the three agents that have been most extensively studied: statins, N-acetylcysteine, and ascorbic acid. Particular attention is paid to the impact of these drugs on the CI-AKI prevention and improved prognosis.

Contrast-induced nephropathy (CIN) is a common condition that is associated with short- and, likely, long-term adverse outcomes. Although periprocedural intravenous hydration is the simplest and most widely used technique to prevent CIN, the limited ability of this approach to mitigate the CIN risk in high-risk populations has provided an impetus to develop new preventive strategies. A range of potentially useful device-based approaches offers new preventive techniques. Well-designed and adequately powered randomized studies of these device-based therapies are urgently needed to determine the expanding role they will play in future clinical practice.

Kidney injury following cardiac catheterization is an infrequent, though persistent, complication, which in some cases may be preventable. Patients at increased risk for renal complications following catheterization can be identified through individual and procedural risk factors, and several risk-prediction models are readily available. The authors advocate for the development of an easily implemented and standardized protocol, readily accessible to catheterization laboratory staff, for the identification and treatment of those patients who may be at increased risk for renal complications following cardiac catheterization.

Surgical or endovascular revascularization procedures for severe peripheral artery disease (PAD) are typically performed in patients with lifestyle-limiting symptoms or evidence of end-organ ischemia secondary to PAD. The role of endovascular therapy in the treatment of PAD is expanding. Contrast-induced nephropathy is the most important and most frequent renal complication of endovascular interventional procedures. Knowledge about complications and their prevention and management is essential for successful outcomes. This article focuses on renal complications during peripheral artery interventions.

Acute kidney injury in hospitalized patients is associated with significantly increased mortality across a broad spectrum of conditions. According to the Society of Thoracic Surgeons database, patients with chronic kidney disease undergoing surgical aortic valve replacement with or without coronary artery bypass grafting had a more than 50% reduction in observed 8-year survival compared with those without chronic kidney disease. Transcatheter aortic valve replacement is an exciting new approach for the treatment of aortic stenosis in high-risk or inoperable patients with severe aortic stenosis. This article discusses the incidence, predictors, impact, and potential avoidance and management strategies of renal dysfunction associated with transcatheter aortic valve replacement.

INTERVENTIONAL CARDIOLOGY CLINICS

Preface
Renal Complications in the Catheterization Laboratory

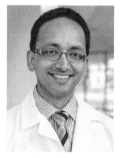 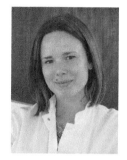

Hitinder S. Gurm, MD   Judith Kooiman, MSc
Editors

Renal disease is of more than a passing interest to the interventional cardiologist. Patients with cardiac disease are more likely to develop renal dysfunction, and those with renal disease are more likely to develop cardiac disease. Renal dysfunction is a major predictor of shorter-term and long-term morbidity and mortality among patients undergoing cardiac interventions. Acute kidney injury (AKI) is a common complication following coronary angiography and intervention and is associated with poor survival. There is great interest in preventing this complication especially since there is no effective treatment other than supportive therapy to manage the complications caused by AKI.

The amount of information provided by the literature on AKI after catheterization is immense and often confusing. An invasive cardiologist is faced with choosing the appropriate prehydration strategy and the safest contrast media and then ensuring that the volume of contrast used is safe. A number of pharmacological approaches have been investigated for the prevention and amelioration of contrast-induced toxicity, and currently, a host of devices are being investigated for this purpose. There is an increasing recognition of AKI among patients undergoing peripheral arterial interventions or those undergoing trans-

catheter aortic valve replacement, although there are only sparse data on the prevention of AKI in this population. This field is rapidly evolving, and a number of innovative tricks and techniques are being explored to limit AKI in these patients.

It is our privilege to present to you an issue of *Interventional Cardiology Clinics* that provides a detailed yet practical overview of the intersection of renal disease and the catheterization laboratory. The authors are internationally recognized experts in this space and have been responsible for leading the key studies that have defined the field. In the initial reviews, they discuss the epidemiology, prediction, and pathophysiology of contrast-induced AKI. Additional articles cover the use of diagnostic biomarkers, differences in nephrotoxicity among contrast agents, the comparative effectiveness of different hydration strategies, and other device and pharmacological preventive measures. Moreover, one article is dedicated to nonrenal complications of iodinated contrast media, as they also occur on a frequent basis, sometimes requiring treatment or prevention in the case of an unavoidable second exposure to iodinated contrast agents.

We would like to thank all the authors who graciously accepted our invitation to contribute to this issue of *Interventional Cardiology Clinics*. We hope that this issue provides relevant and

Intervent Cardiol Clin 3 (2014) xiii–xiv
http://dx.doi.org/10.1016/j.iccl.2014.04.002
2211-7458/14/$ – see front matter © 2014 Elsevier Inc. All rights reserved.

up-to-date perspectives on AKI that you can readily apply in daily practice.

Hitinder S. Gurm, MD
Division of Cardiovascular Medicine
Department of Internal Medicine
Frankel Cardiovascular Center
University of Michigan Health System
University of Michigan Cardiovascular Center
2A394, 1500 E. Medical Center Drive
Ann Arbor, MI 48109-5853, USA

Judith Kooiman, MSc
Departments of Thrombosis and Hemostasis
and Nephrology
Leiden University Medical Center
PO Box 9600, Postal Zone C7-Q
2300 RC Leiden, the Netherlands

E-mail addresses:
hgurm@med.umich.edu (H.S. Gurm)
j.kooiman@lumc.nl (J. Kooiman)

Implications of Kidney Disease in the Cardiac Patient

Roger Rear, BSc, MRCP[a,b], Pascal Meier, MD[a],
Robert M. Bell, BSc, PhD, MRCP[a,b],*

KEYWORDS

- Cardiac • Cardiovascular disease • Chronic kidney disease • Chronic renal failure • Atrial fibrillation
- Coronary artery disease • Chronic heart failure

KEY POINTS

- Chronic kidney disease (CKD) is increasingly prevalent in patients with cardiovascular disease (CVD), and the 2 disease processes are closely interlinked by both etiology and pathophysiology.
- Cardiac patients with CKD may present atypically and have a considerably worse prognosis in all manifestations of CVD, as such, they warrant particularly vigilant specialist treatment.
- There is considerable evidence to support the use of most established cardiac interventions in patients with CKD, although many trials excluded patients with severe CKD and end-stage renal failure.
- Close monitoring of CKD patients is necessary during the treatment of cardiovascular disease to ensure safety and tolerability.

INTRODUCTION

Cardiovascular disease (CVD) and chronic kidney disease (CKD) are both encompassing terms that incorporate a spectrum of pathology that in the case of CVD includes arterial atherosclerosis, heart failure, diseases of the myocardium and pericardium, valvular disease, and cardiac arrhythmias. CKD in turn incorporates vascular, glomerular, tubulointerstitial, and obstructive nephropathies that result in a persistent (minimum of 3 months) depression of glomerular filtration rate (GFR) lower than 90 or, more typically, 60 mL/min/1.73 m^2 (mild and moderate CKD, respectively) and/or the presence of albuminuria. The severity of CKD is classified into 5 categories, as defined by the National Kidney Foundation and the Kidney Disease Outcome Quality Initiative (**Table 1**).[1] Despite the diversity of underlying abnormality in each pathologic condition, there appear to be several etiologic factors shared between CVD and CKD. The noninheritable, noninfectious CVDs typically incorporate "traditional" cardiovascular risk factors that include age, gender, hypertension, diabetes, dyslipidemia, smoking, and other lifestyle factors including obesity. Given that the most common forms of CKD share a significant number of these risk factors, particularly hypertension and diabetes (**Fig. 1**),[2] it is unsurprising that a substantial proportion of cardiac patients also have significant renal impairment: approximately one-third of patients presenting for coronary angiography will have CKD[3–5]; in patients with heart failure the prevalence of CKD is estimated at between 32% and 53% (with the highest prevalence in those with

The authors have nothing to disclose.
[a] General and Interventional Cardiology Department, The Heart Hospital, University College Hospitals NHS Trust, 16-18 Westmoreland Street, London, W1G 8PH, UK; [b] Clinical Research Department, The Hatter Cardiovascular Institute, University College London, 37 Chenies Mews, London, WC1E 6HX, UK
* Corresponding author. The Heart Hospital, University College Hospitals NHS Trust, 16-18 Westmoreland Street, London, W1G 8PH, UK.
E-mail address: rob.bell@ucl.ac.uk

interventional.theclinics.com

Table 1
Classification of chronic kidney disease according to estimated glomerular filtration rate (eGFR)

	eGFR (mL/min/1.73 m²)	Renal Dysfunction	5-Year Mortality (All-Cause) (%)
Stage I	>90	With urine/imaging abnormality	—
Stage II	60–89	Mild	20
Stage IIIa	45–59	Moderate	24
Stage IIIb	34–44	Moderately severe	24
Stage IV	15–29	Severe	46
Stage V	<15	End stage, requiring RRT	55

Mortality data derived from Keith et al,[1] 2004 and US Renal Data System 2013 Annual Data Report.[108]
Abbreviation: RRT, renal replacement therapy.

acute decompensation)[6] and more than half of patients with atrial fibrillation (AF) have CKD,[7] increasing to nearly three-fourths of elderly AF patients (>80 years) considered for anticoagulant therapy.[8]

By contrast, CVDs such as coronary artery disease and heart failure are highly prevalent in the CKD population, and increasingly so with deteriorating renal function: in severe CKD (stage IV), the prevalence of coronary artery disease (CAD) and heart failure reaches 19.0% and 12.5%, respectively.[1] Within this same patient cohort, the prevalence of hypertension and diabetes in individuals with CKD approaches 50% and 20%, respectively. Significantly, these 2 comorbidities represent an increasing worldwide burden: in 2013, 1 billion people were treated for hypertension and 240 million patients for diabetes, with the totals projected to increase to an estimated 1.56 billion with hypertension by 2025 and 380 million with diabetes over the next decade.[2] In these groups, the prevalence of CKD is 37% and 26%, respectively, as reported by the US National Health and

Nutrition Examination Surveys.[9] The prevalence of CKD is therefore anticipated to increase significantly worldwide over the coming decades, and although there have been significant improvements in the rates of cardiovascular mortality (particularly with deaths related to CAD, which have fallen by approximately 50% over the last 3 decades[10]), globally the pressure exerted by increasing prevalence of these comorbidities is contrary to the continuation of this positive trend.

CVD and CKD are intricately linked, and their prognoses interwoven. This review discusses how CKD affects common CVD prognosis, and the efficacy of and the adverse events arising from clinical cardiovascular interventions.

CORONARY ARTERY DISEASE

Atherosclerotic CAD is a prototypical example of the interaction between CKD and CVD. Mild renal dysfunction is increasingly recognized as a nontraditional cardiovascular risk factor for CAD: modest elevations of urinary albumin excretion below the

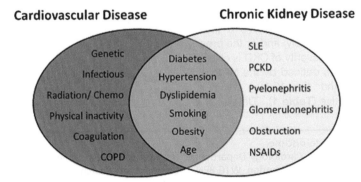

Fig. 1. Significant overlap of risk factors of cardiovascular disease and chronic kidney disease. Venn diagram shows the overlap between the conventional cardiovascular risk factors with the most common causes of chronic kidney disease. Chemo, chemotherapeutic agents used in cancer management; COPD, chronic obstructive pulmonary disease; NSAIDs, nonsteroidal anti-inflammatory drugs; PCKD, polycystic kidney disease; SLE, systemic lupus erythematosus.

current microalbuminemia diagnostic threshold are associated with elevated cardiovascular risk,[11] which increases proportionately with progressive renal deterioration.[12] Moreover, CKD, once established, doubles the rates of both CVD progression[13] and in-hospital death following primary percutaneous intervention (PCI) in comparison with those without CKD.[14] The accelerated progression of CVD in CKD is likely to be multifactorial, incorporating several nontraditional risk factors that include hyperphosphatemia (and vascular calcification),[15] oxidative stress and systemic inflammation,[16] hyperhomocysteinemia, hypervolemia, mineral/electrolyte imbalance, anemia,[17] thrombogenesis, and malnutrition. Consequently, in the CKD patient cohort, CVD mortality is not only 10 to 30 times higher than in the general population,[1] but CVD is a also more likely adverse outcome than progressing to end-stage renal disease (ESRD) in these patients.[18,19] Clinical management strategies therefore must center on the management of the underlying kidney disease and the common causes of hypertension and diabetes; there is emerging evidence that multidisciplinary approaches by nephrologists to control the progression of renal disease pays dividends in diminishing the rates of cardiovascular mortality in these patients.[20]

Difficulties in Diagnosis of Acute Coronary Syndrome

The existence of CKD frequently presents significant diagnostic challenges, not least in the diagnosis of patients presenting with chest pain. The electrocardiogram (ECG) frequently reveals nonspecific abnormalities, so the diagnosis of non–ST-elevation myocardial infarction, a more frequent presentation than ST-elevation myocardial infarction in CKD patients,[21] requires further supportive diagnostic evidence. Patients with CKD frequently have elevated cardiac enzymes on routine testing, which make interpretation of absolute levels problematic, but a change of these cardiac enzymes over a period of 3 to 6 hours will be discriminatory for acute coronary syndrome (ACS).[22] However, persistently elevated cardiac enzymes (such as troponin) should not be ignored in CKD: their elevation is an independent risk factor for cardiovascular mortality.[23] The cause of a chronic troponin increase remains unclear, but is likely to represent myocardial injury potentially relating to microinfarction either secondary to epicardial CAD (53% of patients with advanced CKD will have a coronary stenosis of greater than 50% in 1 or more coronary arteries[24]) or attributable to microvascular dysfunction/left ventricular hypertrophy, with data showing a strong correlation between left ventricular mass and serum troponin levels.[25]

Conversely, the diagnosis of ACS may be missed in patients with CAD and CKD, as the presentation is less likely to be with typical chest pain,[26] potentially reflecting an underlying neuropathy: in the SWEDEHEART register, 67% of CKD patients with ACS had chest pain compared with 90% of those without CKD, and were more likely to present with heart failure.[21] Moreover, more than half of patients referred for renal replacement therapy (RRT) are found to have clinically significant CAD in the absence of characteristic ischemic symptoms.[24]

Noninvasive screening methods for CAD can be used in patients with CKD. CKD patients are vulnerable to calcification of the intima-media of the coronary vessels. Cohort studies have demonstrated CKD to be an independent predictor of high computed tomography (CT) coronary artery calcium (CAC) scores in patients with clinically suspected CAD,[27,28] and CAC scores correlate with the stage of renal dysfunction.[29] Despite debate as to whether CT CAC scores correlate with luminal narrowing, CAC scores are validated as an independent predictor of future cardiac events, correlating with cardiac mortality in CKD patients.[30,31] However, the nephrotoxic risk of contrast exposure in CKD patients has meant that there has been little study of CT–coronary angiography in CKD. Of the other noninvasive screening methods, single-photon emission CT has variable and often low sensitivities in the CKD cohort of patients, and although dobutamine stress echo may be helpful in the screening of CAD, interpretation can prove difficult in the presence of left ventricular hypertrophy frequently found in CKD patients.[32]

Although the diagnosis of CAD in the CKD patient can be problematic, CKD patients have such a high burden of CAD that any cardiovascular presentation should be regarded with considerable suspicion and managed accordingly.[26]

Medical Management of CAD in Patients with CKD

Management of stable CAD consists of a combination of antiplatelet therapy, most commonly with the cyclooxygenase inhibitor aspirin, and aggressive traditional risk-factor management. The coexistence of CKD does not significantly alter this approach.

Aspirin remains beneficial in CKD patients with CAD: in patients with diastolic hypertension, the Hypertension Optimal Treatment (HOT) study found a significant reduction of cardiovascular events, particularly in those with more advanced CKD (IIIb) managed with 75 mg aspirin, compared with control (reduction of major cardiovascular events by two-thirds, overall death reduced by half), with a nonstatistically significant trend toward higher bleeding rates (hazard ratio 2.81, 95% confidence interval [CI] 0.92–8.84, $P = .3$ in the CKD-IIIb group).[33,34]

Reduction of traditional cardiovascular risk factors, particularly hypertension and dyslipidemia, has the potential dual benefit of attenuating the progression of both CVD and CKD. Management of hypertension is well recognized and vital; current guidelines provide a target blood pressure of less than 140/90 mm Hg in the general population, but is amended downward to 130/80 mm Hg in those with CKD.[35] The antihypertensive agents targeting the renin-angiotensin-aldosterone axis, specifically angiotensin-converting enzyme inhibitors (ACE-Is) and angiotensin II receptor blockers (ARBs), are discussed in greater detail in the relevant section herein.

Some controversy has surrounded the effectiveness of 3-hydroxy-3-methyl-glutaryl coenzyme A reductase inhibitors (the statins) in the context of CKD and CAD, but overall the data appear supportive of lipid-lowering agents being helpful in preventing the progression of cardiovascular, if not necessarily renal disease, in both subgroup analysis of existing cardiovascular trials[4] and the prospective Study of Heart and Renal Protection (SHARP).[36] Unfortunately, despite the evident benefit of statin therapy in mild to moderate CKD, statins are disappointingly ineffective in preventing death from CVD in dialysis-dependent end-stage CKD.[37]

β-Blockers for stable angina remain extremely useful in the symptomatic relief of angina symptoms in patients with CKD, but dose adjustments may need to be considered, particularly for the more hydrophilic agents (atenolol, bisoprolol; see later discussion).

In large part the medical management of CAD in patients with CKD is largely unaltered, and the targeting of cardiovascular risk factors benefits both CVD and CKD, with the possible exception of ESRD, in which the protective benefits of statin therapy on CVD seem to be lost.

Implications of CKD and percutaneous coronary intervention

Current interventional guidelines are clear in advocating that ACS management of patients with CKD should not differ from that of patients without.[38] However, it should be recognized that patients with CKD have a worse short-term outcome and a higher adverse event rate, particularly in regard

of major bleeding events, which are nearly double that in the non-CKD population (multivariate odds ratio 1.9, 95% CI 1.22–2.96).[5,39] Great care needs to be invested, therefore, to ensure the use of appropriate doses of renal-excreted antithrombotic drugs, such as enoxaparin, fondaparinux, bivalirudin, and small-molecule glycoprotein IIb/IIIa receptor blockers. In severe CKD these drugs may be contraindicated, and unfractionated heparin used in their place.[38]

A similar pragmatic approach is used in the management of stable CAD. In a post hoc analysis of the Clinical Outcomes Utilizing Revascularization and Aggressive Drug Evaluation (COURAGE) trial comparing outcomes of patients with CKD against those without, both patient groups had similar benefits with identical management strategies. Although PCI conferred no survival benefit in patients with CKD,[40] there was no adverse signal with any combination of PCI and optimal medical therapy, suggesting that these patients should be managed in an individualized fashion comparable with that for non-CKD patients.[41]

In the management of both ACS and stable CAD, there needs to be cognizance of the problems associated with contrast-induced acute kidney injury (CI-AKI). Although CI-AKI is frequently a short-term perturbation of creatinine clearance and is self-limiting, nearly one-fifth of patients may have persistent significant renal impairment[3] and up to 9% will progress to ESRD and dialysis.[42] Current guidelines recommend prehydration, cessation of nephrotoxic agents, and minimization of contrast load,[43] with much current research interest in the potential beneficial roles of high-dose statin[44,45] and remote ischemic conditioning[46,47] as renoprotective strategies during angiographic procedures.

Implication of CKD and coronary artery bypass surgery

Coronary artery bypass grafting (CABG) in patients with CKD, as with PCI, is associated with higher rates of adverse events, particularly for acute kidney injury (25%–40% increase in CKD-III and CKD-IV, respectively)[48] and bleeding events.[49] However, in comparison with PCI in patients with complex, multivessel disease, CABG could be considered as an alternative revascularization strategy. In recent data from large cohort studies, CABG has better cardiovascular outcomes, with lower adjusted mortality, a lower rate of recurrent ACS, and a lower requirement for revascularization when compared with PCI.[50,51] The presence of CKD may also influence decisions regarding the most appropriate surgical approach. In a cohort study of patients undergoing CABG, the off-pump

CABG (OPCAB) group had statistically lower rates of in-hospital mortality and incident RRT in comparison with patients undergoing on-pump CABG (ONCAB), with the strongest effect seen with more advanced renal impairment: unadjusted incidence of mortality in patients with a reduced estimated GFR (eGFR; 15–29 and 30–59 mL/min/1.73 m^2) was lowest among the OPCAB (vs ONCAB) cohort (3.5% vs 5.2% and 2.2% vs 2.4%, respectively), perhaps reflecting an injurious effect of cardiopulmonary bypass and the potential for transient organ hypoperfusion.[52]

Unfortunately there are no data available from large-scale, multicenter, randomized controlled trials to direct clinical management decisions regarding revascularization in high-risk patients with CKD, an area that would certainly benefit from further focused study given the particular problems presented by concomitant multivessel CAD and CKD.

ATRIAL FIBRILLATION

The Framingham Heart Study identified both valvular and nonvalvular risk factors for the development of AF, with significant differences between the genders: men had 50% greater AF prevalence than women, and women were significantly more likely than men to have a valvular etiology. It is recognized that calcific valvular disease is itself associated with CKD, particularly in dialysis-requiring ESRD.[53] Interestingly the major nonvalvular risk factors for the development of AF, in addition to heart failure, are the traditional risk factors for cardiovascular disease, namely age, hypertension, and diabetes.[54] Moreover, CKD is associated with the development of left ventricular hypertrophy, diastolic dysfunction, and subsequent left atrial dilatation,[55] which increases the likelihood of developing AF.[56] Given the risk-factor overlap between CKD and these recognized risk factors for AF, it is not surprising to discover that the prevalence of AF within the CKD cohort of patients is high. In the Chronic Renal Insufficiency Cohort (CRIC) study, the prevalence of AF is 2 to 3 times greater in patients with CKD compared with the general population, with a prevalence of 16% with an eGFR 60 to 45 mL/min/1.73 m^2 rising to more than 20% when the eGFR falls to less than 45 mL/min/1.73 m^2,[57] compared with an estimate of 7.8% in the general population in the REGARDS study.[58] However, whether CKD is a novel AF risk factor is unclear; the increased prevalence of AF within this population may be a simple expression of the presence of several common cardiovascular/renovascular risk factors (hypertension, aging, diabetes) leading to common root disorders such as arterial atherosclerosis, diastolic dysfunction, left ventricular hypertrophy, and heart failure, but the metabolic and electrolyte abnormalities associated with more advanced CKD may nonetheless be unique contributors toward the increased prevalence of AF in the chronic renal impairment cohort.[59]

Impact of CKD on AF Management

In patients with persistent or permanent AF, in whom rate control is the preferred strategy, the use of drugs eliminated from the circulation by the kidney present a particular problem, no more so than for digoxin, which has a narrow therapeutic index and is largely (90%) renally excreted. Indeed, digoxin therapy is associated with a 28% increased risk of death, associated predominantly with toxic digoxin levels and the presence of hypokalemia (a common electrolyte imbalance before dialysis).[60] Other rate-control medications are also not entirely problem-free. β-Blockers as a class have varied excretion: hydrophilic agents such as atenolol and sotolol undergo renal elimination, and these drugs, like those with mixed metabolism such as bisoprolol, will require ECG monitoring and dose adjustments; the best rate-control options in CKD may therefore be lipophilic β-blockers such as metoprolol or carvedilol, or the use of a calcium-channel blocker such as diltiazem.[61] Similarly, in pharmacologic rhythm control strategies, many of the preferred therapy options are limited by their dependence on renal excretion, including sotolol and flecainide (reviewed in Ref.[61]). However, both dronedarone and amiodarone are safe in patients with renal impairment.

Invasive interventions that can potentially cure the arrhythmia are feasible in the context of CKD, and the limitations to drug therapy imposed by CKD seems to make this approach more attractive. However, it should be noted that the success rate of AF ablation in the CKD population is somewhat lower than that found in the general population, with AF recurrence rates after ablation therapy typically 70% greater in CKD patients than in the general population,[62,63] with both low eGFR and left atrial dilatation independently adversely influencing the success of catheter ablation.[64] Therefore, the optimal approaches to the management of AF in CKD patients require the weighing of individual risk factors and outcome benefits. However, as in other areas of CVD in the context of CKD, the main problem in making decisions regarding management of AF in CKD patients is the lack of data from prospective randomized controlled trials.

Impact of CKD on Anticoagulation

Although the inclusion of CKD as a risk factor does not add to the power of the established predictive systemic embolization CHADSVASc[65] risk-scoring system,[66] CKD is nonetheless associated with a significant increase in the risk of thromboembolic stroke arising as a consequence of AF.[67–69] Unfortunately, CKD is also associated with increased bleeding risk, and is recognized in scoring systems such as the HAS-BLED score (Hypertension, Abnormal liver/renal function, Stroke, Bleeding history/predisposition, Labile anticoagulation record, Elderly [>65 years], Drugs/alcohol coadministration/use).[70] Warfarin undergoes hepatic metabolism using the cyp450 enzyme system, although Limdi and colleagues[71] found that warfarin requirements were significantly lower in patients with CKD than in the general population (by 10% and 19% in moderate and severe CKD, respectively). Strict monitoring of the international normalized ratio in patients with CKD is therefore mandatory, and CKD patients without close scrutiny of anticoagulation record suffer high bleeding complication rates, particularly soon after initiation of oral anticoagulant therapy.[72]

There is, however, a general lack of strong data regarding the efficacy of warfarin and its ability to attenuate the rate of thromboembolic stroke in CKD patients, most data being retrospective and nonrandomized.[69,72–75] Moreover, warfarin is associated with vascular calcification related to vitamin K antagonism, and there are reported risks of warfarin-related nephropathy.[61] Despite this, current guidance continues to support the use of anticoagulation for thromboembolic risk reduction in the CKD cohort, which until recently has meant the administration and strict monitoring of warfarin. However, the increasing availability of novel oral anticoagulants will provide greater choice in the management of thromboembolic risk in patients with both AF and CKD. The antithrombin dabigatran[76] and the factor-Xa inhibitors apixaban[77] and rivaroxaban[78] all show at least noninferiority to

warfarin anticoagulation in preventing thromboembolic stroke in mild and moderate CKD patients, with dabigatran and apixaban showing superior systemic embolism risk reduction and dabigatran lower rates of intracranial bleeding when compared with strictly monitored warfarin therapy. Although all 3 of the novel oral anticoagulants have at least an element of renal elimination (dabigatran is 80% renally excreted; the factor-Xa inhibitors less than one-third), all can be used with dose modifications in patients with mild and moderate CKD. None, however, have been trialed in patients with severe CKD and, consequently, only warfarin can be recommended at present for use in patients with an eGFR of less than 15 mL/min/1.73 m^2.

CHRONIC HEART FAILURE

Chronic heart failure (CHF) is a complex clinical syndrome resulting from the inability of the heart to maintain adequate tissue perfusion, because of either structural or functional abnormalities affecting the systolic and/or diastolic phase of the cardiac cycle. CKD is highly prevalent in the CHF patient cohort and, despite the usual exclusion of patients with severe CKD, this is reflected in the landmark heart failure trial literature, with prevalence rates estimated between 32% and 50% (Table 2). CKD adversely affects the prognosis of CHF: a recent meta-analysis of 85 CHF trials (comprising 49,890 patients) revealed a doubling of all-cause mortality within this patient population (Table 3).[6]

The link between CHF and CKD is in part attributable to shared etiologic risk factors, but is also a direct consequence of the interaction of their respective pathophysiology (Fig. 2). For example, low cardiac output and increased venous congestion (predominant in heart failure with preserved ejection fraction) respectively reduce renal arterial blood flow and perfusion gradient,[79] exacerbating kidney dysfunction, which can be further aggravated by the therapies used to manage CHF, through any combination of diuresis-associated

Table 2
Prevalence of CKD by major CHF trial

Study	Treatment	Exclusion Creatinine (μmol/L)	CKD Prevalence (%) eGFR <60 mL/min/1.73 m^2
SOLVD[109]	Enalapril	>177	32
CHARM[110]	Candesartan	>265	36
CIBIS-II[81]	Bisoprolol	>300	33
CARE-HF[111]	CRT	N/A	50

Abbreviations: CHF, chronic heart failure; CKD, chronic kidney disease; CRT, cardiac resynchronization therapy; eGFR, estimated glomerular filtration rate; N/A, no data available.

Table 3
All-cause mortality based on severity of CKD

	All CKD 32% Prevalence	Moderate CKD	Severe CKD	WRF 23% Prevalence
All-cause mortality	2.34 OR 95% CI 2.2–2.5 P<.001	1.59 HR 95% CI 1.49–1.69 P<.001	2.17 HR 95% CI 1.95–2.40 P<.001	1.81 OR 95% CI 1.55–2.12 P<.001

Abbreviations: CI, confidence interval; CKD, chronic kidney disease; HR, hazard ratio; OR, odds ratio; WRF, worsening renal function.

Data from Damman K, Valente MA, Voors AA, et al. Renal impairment, worsening renal function, and outcome in patients with heart failure: an updated meta-analysis. Eur Heart J 2014;35(7):455–69.

hypovolemia, renin-angiotensin-aldosterone system (RAAS) inhibitors, and drug-induced hypotension. By contrast, renal dysfunction leads to neurohormonal dysregulation, anemia, volume overload, and complex inflammatory cascades that negatively affect cardiac function. The bidirectional interaction between 2 failing organ systems can lead to a vicious cycle of progressive cardiac and renal dysfunction, termed cardiorenal syndrome, the classifications of which are summarized in **Table 4**.[80]

Medical Management of CHF in Patients with CKD

The established canon of CHF management consists of ACE-Is/ARBs, β-blockers, and mineralocorticoid receptor antagonists (MRAs), with 2 decades of landmark mortality outcome data to support their use (**Table 5**). In patients with normal renal function, all improve prognosis, reduce hospitalizations, and improve mortality rates. The coexistence of CKD, however, introduces particular challenges for the introduction and maintenance of CHF therapy.

Perhaps the most innocuous of these drug classes are the β-blockers. β-Blockers have no adverse impact on the progression of CKD, and the efficacy of β-blockade in CHF seems unaltered by the existence of CKD: a retrospective analysis of outcomes in the CIBIS-II study reported preserved relative risk reduction in patients treated with bisoprolol at all stages of CKD,[81] data supported from observations in the MERIT-HF trial.[82] As discussed earlier, individual β-blockers have variable dependence on renal elimination: hydrophilic drugs (atenolol and bisoprolol) will require dose adjustments and monitoring in CKD, whereas the lipophilic β-blockers (carvedilol and metoprolol), which undergo hepatic metabolism, do not,[83] an observation that may help influence the optimal choice of therapeutic agent.

By contrast, drugs that affect the RAAS axis require greater caution when CHF coexists with CKD. The ACE-Is/ARBs are a prototypical example of this. In addition to their role in the management of CHF, ACE-Is and ARBs are also pivotal to the management of CKD, attenuating progression of hypertensive, proteinuric CKD[84] and lower mortality rates, as suggested by retrospective population studies.[85] However ACE-Is/ARBs are not innocuous in terms of renal function: a modest perturbation of GFR is frequently found following ACE-I or ARB initiation, with an increase of creatinine to a new 10- to 20-μmol/L higher baseline observed in the CONSENSUS study.[86] However, although

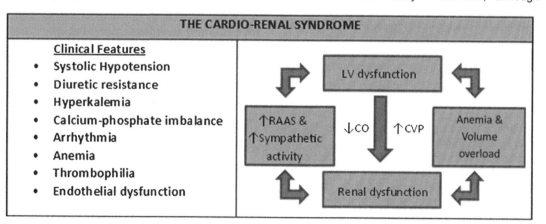

Fig. 2. The cardiorenal syndrome: clinical features and pathophysiologic mechanism. CO, cardiac output; CVP, central venous pressure; LV, left ventricle; RAAS, renin-angiotensin-aldosterone system.

Table 4
Cardiorenal syndrome classification system adopted at the 2010 ADQI consensus conference

Type	Inciting Event	Secondary Disturbance	Example
Type 1 Acute cardiorenal syndrome	Abrupt worsening of cardiac function	Acute kidney injury	Acute cardiogenic shock or acute decompensation of chronic heart failure
Type 2 Chronic cardiorenal syndrome	Chronic abnormalities in cardiac function	Chronic kidney damage	Chronic heart failure
Type 3 Acute renocardiac syndrome	Abrupt worsening of renal function	Acute cardiac dysfunction (eg, heart failure or arrhythmia)	Acute kidney injury or glomerular nephritis
Type 4 Chronic renocardiac syndrome	Chronic kidney disease	Decreased cardiac function, cardiac hypertrophy, and/or increased risk of adverse cardiovascular events	Chronic glomerular disease
Type 5 Secondary cardiorenal syndrome	Systemic disease	Cardiac and renal dysfunction	Diabetes mellitus, systemic lupus, sepsis, etc

Cardiorenal syndromes are divided into 5 categories according to triggering event and its consequence.
Abbreviation: ADQI, Acute Dialysis Quality Initiative.
Adapted from Ronco C, McCullough P, Anker SD, et al. Cardio-renal syndromes: report from the consensus conference of the acute dialysis quality initiative. Eur Heart J 2010;31:703–11.

CHF studies excluded patients with severe CKD, in patients with mild and moderate CKD the cardiovascular mortality benefit of ACE-Is/ARBs appears to be preserved.[87–89]

With respect to the MRAs, both the RALES[90] and EMPHASIS-HF studies[91] (in which half and a third of patients had CKD, respectively) demonstrated mortality reductions (30% and 34%, respectively), in addition to reduced symptoms and hospitalizations. Both trials excluded patients with severe CKD (RALES used a cutoff of 221 mmol/L; EMPHASIS-HF an eGFR of 30 mL/min/1.73 m²), but MRAs remain effective therapies in CHF when there is coexistent mild to moderate CKD.[92] Unfortunately, the use of aldosterone antagonists in patients with severe CKD can provoke hyperkalemia, especially in conjunction with ACE-Is or ARBs. Current European guidelines recommend that a serum creatinine level higher than 220 µmol/L or potassium level higher than 5 mmol/L is a contraindication, although cautious use is usually well tolerated in mild or moderate CKD.[93]

Excessive sodium and water retention is usually present in CHF patients with CKD, and should be treated initially with dietary sodium restriction (<2 g salt/d), but may require intensive diuretic therapy using the minimum dose required to achieve a "dry weight"; diuretic overdosing is associated with increased mortality.[94] Loop diuretics are more effective than thiazide diuretics, and, if necessary, cautious combination of both agents may be used.[95] However, unlike the MRA class of diuretics, there is no prognostic benefit to be derived from loop or thiazide diuretics in the setting of either CHF or CKD.

Management of Anemia

Anemia is a significant problem in patients with CHF and CKD, and often remains overlooked in busy specialist clinics.[96] CHF mortality increases with severity of anemia by 50% to 100%[97] and the presence of CKD further doubles the mortality.[98] Current European guidelines recommend correcting hemoglobin levels to between 10 and 12 g/dL; however, recent systematic reviews and meta-analyses have shown worse outcomes when levels are normalized (>13 g/dL).[99,100] Initial correction of iron deficiency with oral or parenteral iron before low-dose erythropoietin-stimulating agents are recommended to minimize the need for blood transfusions.

Device Therapy

Post hoc subanalysis of CARE-HF[101] showed that the relative effect of cardiac resynchronization therapy (CRT) was similar among eGFR subgroups, whereas subanalysis of the MIRACLE

Table 5
Summary of the major CHF trials with CKD subgroup analysis data

Trial Name	Treatment/Target (Mean Daily Dose)	Outcome	Effect (%)	CKD I–III Effect	CKD IV–V Effect
CONSENSUS[112]	Enalapril 20 mg bid (18.4 mg)	1°: All-cause mortality	RRR 27, ARR 15	Preserved	Preserved (NS) <30 mL/min/1.73 m²
SOLVD[109]	Enalapril 10 mg bid (16.6 mg)	1°: All-cause mortality	RRR 16	Preserved	Preserved <45 mL/min/1.73 m²
CHARM-ALT[110]	Candesartan 32 mg qd (23 mg)	1°: CV mortality + HF admission	RRR 23, AR 7	Preserved	No data
MERIT-HF[113]	Metoprolol 200 mg qd (159 mg)	1°: All-cause mortality	RRR 34, ARR 3.8	Preserved	Preserved <45 mL/min/1.73 m²
CIBIS-II[114]	Bisoprolol 10 mg qd (8.6 mg)	1°: All-cause mortality	RRR 32, ARR 5.5	Preserved	Preserved <45 mL/min/1.73 m²
COPERNICUS[115] CAPRICORN[116]	Carvedilol 25 mg bid (37 mg)	1°: All-cause mortality	RRR 35, ARR 5.6	Preserved	Preserved <45 mL/min/1.73 m²
RALES[90]	Spironolactone 50 mg qd (26 mg)	1°: All-cause mortality	RRR 30, ARR 11	Preserved	Contraindicated
EMPHASIS-HF[91]	Eplerenone 50 mg qd (39.1 mg), 25 mg CKD III	1°: CV mortality + HF admission	RRR 34, ARR 7.6	Preserved	Contraindicated
DIG[117]	Digoxin variable (0.25 mg)	2°: HF admission	RRR 28, ARR 7.9	Preserved	Preserved
SHIFT[118]	Ivabradine 7.5 mg bid (6.5 mg)	1°: CV mortality+ HF admission	RRR 18, ARR 5	No data	No data
A-HEFT[119]	Hydralazine/ISDN 75 mg/40 mg tid (142.5 mg/76 mg)	1°: All-cause mortality + HF admission + QOL	RRR 43[a]/33[b], ARR 4.0[a]/8[b]	No data	No data
MADIT II[120]	ICD	1°: All-cause mortality	RRR 31, ARR 5.6	Preserved	Preserved (NS)
CARE-HF[111]	CRT	1°: CV mortality + CV admission	RRR 37, ARR 16	Preserved	No data
MADIT-CRT[121]	CRT-D	1°: All-cause mortality + HF admission	RRR 17.2, ARR 8.1	Preserved	No data

Abbreviations: ARR, absolute risk reduction; bid, twice daily; CRT, cardiac resynchronization therapy; CRT-D, cardiac resynchronization therapy with defibrillation; CV, cardiovascular; HF, heart failure; ICD, implantable cardioverter-defibrillator; ISDN, isosorbide dinitrate; NS, not significant; qd, once daily; QOL, quality of life score; RRR, relative risk reduction; tid, 3 times daily.

[a] All-Cause Mortality.
[b] Heart Failure admission.

study demonstrated an improvement in baseline renal function.[102] However, another subanalysis of the REVERSE study[103] found that CKD patients treated with CRT had worse left ventricular parameter outcomes, which the investigators attributed to CKD-specific impairment of reverse left ventricular remodeling. For patients who might reasonably be expected to proceed to dialysis, consideration of the site of arteriovenous fistula before device implantation is recommended to avoid complications secondary to pacing wire–associated central venous stenosis.[104]

Patients with CKD have a significantly increased risk of sudden cardiac death (SCD) from ventricular arrhythmia, particularly so during dialysis, and limited evidence suggests they should be offered implantable cardioverter-defibrillator (ICD) therapy if they meet the usual criteria[105]; however, concerns exist regarding the efficacy of ICDs in ESRD.[106] Unfortunately, SCD during dialysis may occur in the absence of typical ICD criteria, owing to complex interactions between hemodynamic, electrolytic, hypertrophic, and electrophysiologic factors,[107] and further prospective studies are required before any specific recommendations can be made.

SUMMARY

Renal disease is a frequent partner of cardiovascular disease, whereby the presence of one accelerates the progression of the other. Moreover, renal disease adversely affects the efficacy and tolerability of a range of medical, interventional, and surgical interventions in CVD. Overall, however, the basic tenets of cardiovascular management remain unchanged by the presence of renal disease, no matter how advanced. Treatment priorities remain the early identification of risk factors, treatment and prevention of CKD and CVD where possible, and, where present, attenuation of the progression of both disease states. Moreover, clinicians should avoid the occurrence of acute kidney injury, through the use of drugs such as ACE-Is, or the minimization of hypotension, nephrotoxics, or contrast agents during invasive or surgical procedures. A key problem in the management of patients with CKD is the lack of prospective, randomized controlled trials. Data from such studies are sorely needed in a variety of areas such as the optimum strategy in patients with moderate and severe CKD and concomitant CAD, CHF, or AF. Therefore, more extensive study is required in this area of cardiovascular medicine to broaden the understanding of the underlying disease processes and to validate medical interventions from drugs through to surgery in the context of kidney impairment, thus ensuring optimal outcomes and preservation of quality of life in this challenging patient cohort.

REFERENCES

1. Keith DS, Nichols GA, Gullion CM, et al. Longitudinal follow-up and outcomes among a population with chronic kidney disease in a large managed care organization. Arch Intern Med 2004;164:659–63.
2. Bakris GL, Ritz E. The message for world kidney day 2009: hypertension and kidney disease: a marriage that should be prevented. Kidney Int 2009; 75:449–52.
3. Maioli M, Toso A, Leoncini M, et al. Persistent renal damage after contrast-induced acute kidney injury:
4. incidence, evolution, risk factors, and prognosis. Circulation 2012;125:3099–107.
4. Shepherd J, Kastelein JJ, Bittner V, et al. Intensive lipid lowering with atorvastatin in patients with coronary heart disease and chronic kidney disease: the TNT (treating to new targets) study. J Am Coll Cardiol 2008;51:1448–54.
5. Santopinto JJ, Fox KA, Goldberg RJ, et al. Creatinine clearance and adverse hospital outcomes in patients with acute coronary syndromes: findings from the global registry of acute coronary events (grace). Heart 2003;89:1003–8.
6. Damman K, Valente MA, Voors AA, et al. Renal impairment, worsening renal function, and outcome in patients with heart failure: an updated meta-analysis. Eur Heart J 2014;35:455–69.
7. Hohnloser SH, Hijazi Z, Thomas L, et al. Efficacy of apixaban when compared with warfarin in relation to renal function in patients with atrial fibrillation: insights from the ARISTOTLE trial. Eur Heart J 2012; 33:2821–30.
8. Poli D, Antonucci E, Zanazzi M, et al. Impact of glomerular filtration estimate on bleeding risk in very old patients treated with vitamin k antagonists. Results of EPICA study on the behalf of FCSA (Italian Federation of Anticoagulation Clinics). Thromb Haemost 2012;107:1100–6.
9. Ostchega Y, Yoon SS, Hughes J, et al. Hypertension awareness, treatment, and control—continued disparities in adults: United States, 2005-2006. NCHS Data Brief 2008;1–8.
10. Nichols M, Townsend N, Scarborough P, et al. Trends in age-specific coronary heart disease mortality in the European Union over three decades: 1980-2009. Eur Heart J 2013;34:3017–27.
11. Cerasola G, Cottone S, Mule G. The progressive pathway of microalbuminuria: from early marker of renal damage to strong cardiovascular risk predictor. J Hypertens 2010;28:2357–69.
12. Vanholder R, Massy Z, Argiles A, et al. Chronic kidney disease as cause of cardiovascular morbidity and mortality. Nephrol Dial Transplant 2005;20: 1048–56.
13. Collins AJ, Li S, Gilbertson DT, et al. Chronic kidney disease and cardiovascular disease in the Medicare population. Kidney Int Suppl 2003;64(Suppl 87): S24–31.
14. Gevaert SA, De Bacquer D, Evrard P, et al. Renal dysfunction in STEMI-patients undergoing primary angioplasty: higher prevalence but equal prognostic impact in female patients; an observational cohort study from the Belgian STEMI Registry. BMC Nephrol 2013;14:62.
15. Kanbay M, Goldsmith D, Akcay A, et al. Phosphate—the silent stealthy cardiorenal culprit in all stages of chronic kidney disease: a systematic review. Blood Purif 2009;27:220–30.

16. Cachofeiro V, Goicochea M, de Vinuesa SG, et al. Oxidative stress and inflammation, a link between chronic kidney disease and cardiovascular disease. Kidney Int Suppl 2008;74(Suppl 111):S4–9.

17. McCullough PA, Lepor NE. Piecing together the evidence on anemia: the link between chronic kidney disease and cardiovascular disease. Rev Cardiovasc Med 2005;6(Suppl 3):S4–12.

18. Shulman NB, Ford CE, Hall WD, et al. Prognostic value of serum creatinine and effect of treatment of hypertension on renal function. Results from the hypertension detection and follow-up program. The Hypertension Detection and Follow-Up Program Cooperative Group. Hypertension 1989;13:l80–93.

19. Berl T, Henrich W. Kidney-heart interactions: epidemiology, pathogenesis, and treatment. Clin J Am Soc Nephrol 2006;1:8–18.

20. Luciano Ede P, Luconi PS, Sesso RC, et al. Prospective study of 2151 patients with chronic kidney disease under conservative treatment with multidisciplinary care in the Vale do Paraiba, SP. J Bras Nefrol 2012;34:226–34.

21. Szummer K, Lundman P, Jacobson SH, et al. Relation between renal function, presentation, use of therapies and in-hospital complications in acute coronary syndrome: data from the Swedeheart Register. J Intern Med 2010;268:40–9.

22. Thygesen K, Alpert JS, Jaffe AS, et al. Third universal definition of myocardial infarction. J Am Coll Cardiol 2012;60:1581–98.

23. End C, Seliger SL, Defilippi CR. Interpreting cardiac troponin results from highly sensitive assays in patients with chronic kidney disease: acute coronary syndromes and beyond. Coron Artery Dis 2013;24:720–3.

24. Ohtake T, Kobayashi S, Moriya H, et al. High prevalence of occult coronary artery stenosis in patients with chronic kidney disease at the initiation of renal replacement therapy: an angiographic examination. J Am Soc Nephrol 2005;16:1141–8.

25. Iliou MC, Fumeron C, Benoit MO, et al. Factors associated with increased serum levels of cardiac troponins T and I in chronic haemodialysis patients: Chronic Haemodialysis and New Cardiac Markers Evaluation (CHANCE) study. Nephrol Dial Transplant 2001;16:1452–8.

26. Komukai K, Ogawa T, Yagi H, et al. Renal insufficiency is related to painless myocardial infarction. Circ J 2007;71:1366–9.

27. Kramer H, Toto R, Peshock R, et al. Association between chronic kidney disease and coronary artery calcification: the Dallas Heart Study. J Am Soc Nephrol 2005;16:507–13.

28. Cao XF, Yan LQ, Han LX, et al. Association of mild to moderate kidney dysfunction with coronary artery calcification in patients with suspected coronary artery disease. Cardiology 2011;120:211–6.

29. Budoff MJ, Rader DJ, Reilly MP, et al. Relationship of estimated GFR and coronary artery calcification in the CRIC (Chronic Renal Insufficiency Cohort) study. Am J Kidney Dis 2011;58:519–26.

30. Chiu YW, Adler SG, Budoff MJ, et al. Coronary artery calcification and mortality in diabetic patients with proteinuria. Kidney Int 2010;77:1107–14.

31. Russo D, Morrone L, Russo L. Coronary artery calcification and cardiovascular mortality in predialysis patients. Kidney Int 2011;79:258 [author reply: 258].

32. Karthikeyan V, Ananthasubramaniam K. Coronary risk assessment and management options in chronic kidney disease patients prior to kidney transplantation. Curr Cardiol Rev 2009;5:177–86.

33. Hansson L, Zanchetti A, Carruthers SG, et al. Effects of intensive blood-pressure lowering and low-dose aspirin in patients with hypertension: principal results of the Hypertension Optimal Treatment (HOT) randomised trial. HOT Study Group. Lancet 1998;351:1755–62.

34. Jardine MJ, Ninomiya T, Perkovic V, et al. Aspirin is beneficial in hypertensive patients with chronic kidney disease: a post-hoc subgroup analysis of a randomized controlled trial. J Am Coll Cardiol 2010;56:956–65.

35. Rosendorff C. Hypertension and coronary artery disease: a summary of the American Heart Association scientific statement. J Clin Hypertens (Greenwich) 2007;9:790–5.

36. Baigent C, Landray MJ, Reith C, et al. The effects of lowering LDL cholesterol with simvastatin plus ezetimibe in patients with chronic kidney disease (Study of Heart and Renal Protection): a randomised placebo-controlled trial. Lancet 2011;377:2181–92.

37. Wanner C, Krane V, Marz W, et al. Atorvastatin in patients with type 2 diabetes mellitus undergoing hemodialysis. N Engl J Med 2005;353:238–48.

38. Hamm CW, Bassand JP, Agewall S, et al. ESC guidelines for the management of acute coronary syndromes in patients presenting without persistent ST-segment elevation: the Task Force for the Management of Acute Coronary Syndromes (ACS) in patients presenting without persistent ST-segment elevation of the European Society of Cardiology (ESC). Eur Heart J 2011;32:2999–3054.

39. Moscucci M, Fox KA, Cannon CP, et al. Predictors of major bleeding in acute coronary syndromes: the Global Registry of Acute Coronary Events (GRACE). Eur Heart J 2003;24:1815–23.

40. Sedlis SP, Jurkovitz CT, Hartigan PM, et al. Optimal medical therapy with or without percutaneous coronary intervention for patients with stable coronary artery disease and chronic kidney disease. Am J Cardiol 2009;104:1647–53.

41. Sedlis SP, Jurkovitz CT, Hartigan PM, et al. Health status and quality of life in patients with stable coronary artery disease and chronic kidney disease treated with optimal medical therapy or percutaneous coronary intervention (post hoc findings from the COURAGE trial). Am J Cardiol 2013;112:1703–8.

42. Reed M, Meier P, Tamhane UU, et al. The relative renal safety of iodixanol compared with low-osmolar contrast media: a meta-analysis of randomized controlled trials. JACC Cardiovasc Interv 2009;2:645–54.

43. Hecker PA, Leopold JA, Gupte SA, et al. Impact of glucose-6-phosphate dehydrogenase deficiency on the pathophysiology of cardiovascular disease. Am J Physiol Heart Circ Physiol 2013;304:H491–500.

44. Leoncini M, Toso A, Maioli M, et al. Early high-dose rosuvastatin for contrast-induced nephropathy prevention in acute coronary syndrome. Results from Protective Effect of Rosuvastatin and Antiplatelet Therapy on Contrast-Induced Acute Kidney Injury and Myocardial Damage in Patients with Acute Coronary Syndrome (PRATO-ACS study). J Am Coll Cardiol 2013;63:71–9.

45. Hoshi T, Sato A, Kakefuda Y, et al. Preventive effect of statin pretreatment on contrast-induced acute kidney injury in patients undergoing coronary angioplasty: propensity score analysis from a multicenter registry. Int J Cardiol 2014;171:243–9.

46. Er F, Nia AM, Dopp H, et al. Ischemic preconditioning for prevention of contrast medium-induced nephropathy: randomized pilot RENPRO trial (renal protection trial). Circulation 2012;126:296–303.

47. Deftereos S, Giannopoulos G, Tzalamouras V, et al. Renoprotective effect of remote ischemic post-conditioning by intermittent balloon inflations in patients undergoing percutaneous coronary intervention. J Am Coll Cardiol 2013;61:1949–55.

48. Huang TM, Wu VC, Young GH, et al. Preoperative proteinuria predicts adverse renal outcomes after coronary artery bypass grafting. J Am Soc Nephrol 2011;22:156–63.

49. Winkelmayer WC, Levin R, Avorn J. Chronic kidney disease as a risk factor for bleeding complications after coronary artery bypass surgery. Am J Kidney Dis 2003;41:84–9.

50. Chang TI, Leong TK, Kazi DS, et al. Comparative effectiveness of coronary artery bypass grafting and percutaneous coronary intervention for multivessel coronary disease in a community-based population with chronic kidney disease. Am Heart J 2013;165:800–8, 808.e1–2.

51. Weintraub WS, Grau-Sepulveda MV, Weiss JM, et al. Comparative effectiveness of revascularization strategies. N Engl J Med 2012;366:1467–76.

52. Chawla LS, Zhao Y, Lough FC, et al. Off-pump versus on-pump coronary artery bypass grafting outcomes stratified by preoperative renal function. J Am Soc Nephrol 2012;23:1389–97.

53. Umana E, Ahmed W, Alpert MA. Valvular and perivalvular abnormalities in end-stage renal disease. Am J Med Sci 2003;325:237–42.

54. Benjamin EJ, Levy D, Vaziri SM, et al. Independent risk factors for atrial fibrillation in a population-based cohort. The Framingham Heart Study. JAMA 1994;271:840–4.

55. Cerasola G, Nardi E, Palermo A, et al. Epidemiology and pathophysiology of left ventricular abnormalities in chronic kidney disease: a review. J Nephrol 2011;24:1–10.

56. Wachtell K, Devereux RB, Lyle PA, et al. The left atrium, atrial fibrillation, and the risk of stroke in hypertensive patients with left ventricular hypertrophy. Ther Adv Cardiovasc Dis 2008;2:507–13.

57. Soliman EZ, Prineas RJ, Go AS, et al. Chronic kidney disease and prevalent atrial fibrillation: the Chronic Renal Insufficiency Cohort (CRIC). Am Heart J 2010;159:1102–7.

58. Prineas RJ, Soliman EZ, Howard G, et al. The sensitivity of the method used to detect atrial fibrillation in population studies affects group-specific prevalence estimates: ethnic and regional distribution of atrial fibrillation in the regards study. J Epidemiol 2009;19:177–81.

59. Korantzopoulos P, Liu T, Letsas KP, et al. The epidemiology of atrial fibrillation in end-stage renal disease. J Nephrol 2013;26:617–23.

60. Chan KE, Lazarus JM, Hakim RM. Digoxin associates with mortality in ESRD. J Am Soc Nephrol 2010;21:1550–9.

61. Nimmo C, Wright M, Goldsmith D. Management of atrial fibrillation in chronic kidney disease: double trouble. Am Heart J 2013;166:230–9.

62. Berkowitsch A, Kuniss M, Greiss H, et al. Impact of impaired renal function and metabolic syndrome on the recurrence of atrial fibrillation after catheter ablation: a long term follow-up. Pacing Clin Electrophysiol 2012;35:532–43.

63. Naruse Y, Tada H, Sekiguchi Y, et al. Concomitant chronic kidney disease increases the recurrence of atrial fibrillation after catheter ablation of atrial fibrillation: a mid-term follow-up. Heart Rhythm 2011;8:335–41.

64. Tokuda M, Yamane T, Matsuo S, et al. Relationship between renal function and the risk of recurrent atrial fibrillation following catheter ablation. Heart 2011;97:137–42.

65. Lip GY, Nieuwlaat R, Pisters R, et al. Refining clinical risk stratification for predicting stroke and thromboembolism in atrial fibrillation using a novel risk factor-based approach: the Euro

Heart Survey on Atrial Fibrillation. Chest 2010; 137:263–72.

66. Roldan V, Marin F, Manzano-Fernandez S, et al. Does chronic kidney disease improve the predictive value of the CHADS2 and CHA2DS2-VASC stroke stratification risk scores for atrial fibrillation? Thromb Haemost 2013;109:956–60.

67. Go AS, Fang MC, Udaltsova N, et al. Impact of proteinuria and glomerular filtration rate on risk of thromboembolism in atrial fibrillation: the Anticoagulation and Risk Factors in Atrial Fibrillation (ATRIA) study. Circulation 2009;119:1363–9.

68. Nakagawa K, Hirai T, Takashima S, et al. Chronic kidney disease and CHADS(2) score independently predict cardiovascular events and mortality in patients with nonvalvular atrial fibrillation. Am J Cardiol 2011;107:912–6.

69. Olesen JB, Lip GY, Kamper AL, et al. Stroke and bleeding in atrial fibrillation with chronic kidney disease. N Engl J Med 2012;367:625–35.

70. Pisters R, Lane DA, Nieuwlaat R, et al. A novel user-friendly score (has-bled) to assess 1-year risk of major bleeding in patients with atrial fibrillation: The Euro Heart Survey. Chest 2010;138:1093–100.

71. Limdi NA, Limdi MA, Cavallari L, et al. Warfarin dosing in patients with impaired kidney function. Am J Kidney Dis 2010;56:823–31.

72. Chan KE, Lazarus JM, Thadhani R, et al. Warfarin use associates with increased risk for stroke in hemodialysis patients with atrial fibrillation. J Am Soc Nephrol 2009;20:2223–33.

73. Winkelmayer WC, Liu J, Setoguchi S, et al. Effectiveness and safety of warfarin initiation in older hemodialysis patients with incident atrial fibrillation. Clin J Am Soc Nephrol 2011;6:2662–8.

74. Lai HM, Aronow WS, Kalen P, et al. Incidence of thromboembolic stroke and of major bleeding in patients with atrial fibrillation and chronic kidney disease treated with and without warfarin. Int J Nephrol Renovasc Dis 2009;2:33–7.

75. Knoll F, Sturm G, Lamina C, et al. Coumarins and survival in incident dialysis patients. Nephrol Dial Transplant 2012;27:332–7.

76. Connolly SJ, Ezekowitz MD, Yusuf S, et al. Dabigatran versus warfarin in patients with atrial fibrillation. N Engl J Med 2009;361:1139–51.

77. Granger CB, Alexander JH, McMurray JJ, et al. Apixaban versus warfarin in patients with atrial fibrillation. N Engl J Med 2011;365:981–92.

78. Patel MR, Mahaffey KW, Garg J, et al. Rivaroxaban versus warfarin in nonvalvular atrial fibrillation. N Engl J Med 2011;365:883–91.

79. Damman K, Navis G, Smilde TD, et al. Decreased cardiac output, venous congestion and the association with renal impairment in patients with cardiac dysfunction. Eur J Heart Fail 2007;9:872–8.

80. Brown JR, Uber PA, Mehra MR. The progressive cardiorenal syndrome in heart failure: Mechanisms and therapeutic insights. Curr Treat Options Cardiovasc Med 2008;10:342–8.

81. Erdmann E, Lechat P, Verkenne P, et al. Results from post-hoc analyses of the CIBIS II trial: effect of bisoprolol in high-risk patient groups with chronic heart failure. Eur J Heart Fail 2001;3:469–79.

82. Ghali JK, Wikstrand J, Van Veldhuisen DJ, et al. The influence of renal function on clinical outcome and response to beta-blockade in systolic heart failure: insights from Metoprolol CR/XL Randomized Intervention Trial in Chronic HF (MERIT-HF). J Card Fail 2009;15:310–8.

83. Bakris GL, Hart P, Ritz E. Beta blockers in the management of chronic kidney disease. Kidney Int 2006;70:1905–13.

84. Sarafidis PA, Ruilope LM. Aggressive blood pressure reduction and renin-angiotensin system blockade in chronic kidney disease: time for re-evaluation? Kidney Int 2013;85:536–46.

85. Molnar MZ, Kalantar-Zadeh K, Lott EH, et al. ACE inhibitor and angiotensin receptor blocker use and mortality in patients with chronic kidney disease. J Am Coll Cardiol 2014;63(7):650–8.

86. Ljungman S, Kjekshus J, Swedberg K. Renal function in severe congestive heart failure during treatment with enalapril (the Cooperative North Scandinavian Enalapril Survival Study [Consensus] Trial). Am J Cardiol 1992;70:479–87.

87. Swedberg K, Eneroth P, Kjekshus J, et al. Effects of enalapril and neuroendocrine activation on prognosis in severe congestive heart failure (follow-up of the Consensus Trial). Consensus Trial Study Group. Am J Cardiol 1990;66:40D–4D [discussion: 44D–45D].

88. Bowling CB, Sanders PW, Allman RM, et al. Effects of enalapril in systolic heart failure patients with and without chronic kidney disease: insights from the SOLVD treatment trial. Int J Cardiol 2013;167: 151–6.

89. Konstam MA, Neaton JD, Dickstein K, et al. Effects of high-dose versus low-dose losartan on clinical outcomes in patients with heart failure (HEAAL study): a randomised, double-blind trial. Lancet 2009;374:1840–8.

90. Pitt B, Zannad F, Remme WJ, et al. The effect of spironolactone on morbidity and mortality in patients with severe heart failure. Randomized Aldactone Evaluation Study Investigators. N Engl J Med 1999;341:709–17.

91. Zannad F, McMurray JJ, Krum H, et al. Eplerenone in patients with systolic heart failure and mild symptoms. N Engl J Med 2011;364:11–21.

92. Vardeny O, Wu DH, Desai A, et al, RALES Investigators. Influence of baseline and worsening renal

function on efficacy of spironolactone in patients with severe heart failure: insights from RALES (Randomized Aldactone Evaluation Study). J Am Coll Cardiol 2012;60:2082–9.

93. McMurray JJ, Adamopoulos S, Anker SD, et al, Task Force for the Diagnosis and Treatment of Acute and Chronic Heart Failure of the European Society of Cardiology, Guidelines ESC Committee for Practice. ESC guidelines for the diagnosis and treatment of acute and chronic heart failure 2012: the Task Force for the Diagnosis and Treatment of Acute and Chronic Heart Failure 2012 of the European Society of Cardiology. Developed in collaboration with the Heart Failure Association (HFA) of the ESC. Eur J Heart Fail 2012;14:803–69.

94. Eshaghian S, Horwich TB, Fonarow GC. Relation of loop diuretic dose to mortality in advanced heart failure. Am J Cardiol 2006;97:1759–64.

95. Wollam GL, Tarazi RC, Bravo EL, et al. Diuretic potency of combined hydrochlorothiazide and furosemide therapy in patients with azotemia. Am J Med 1982;72:929–38.

96. Tang WH, Tong W, Jain A, et al. Evaluation and long-term prognosis of new-onset, transient, and persistent anemia in ambulatory patients with chronic heart failure. J Am Coll Cardiol 2008;51:569–76.

97. Kosiborod M, Smith GL, Radford MJ, et al. The prognostic importance of anemia in patients with heart failure. Am J Med 2003;114:112–9.

98. Al-Ahmad A, Rand WM, Manjunath G, et al. Reduced kidney function and anemia as risk factors for mortality in patients with left ventricular dysfunction. J Am Coll Cardiol 2001;38:955–62.

99. Palmer SC, Navaneethan SD, Craig JC, et al. Meta-analysis: erythropoiesis-stimulating agents in patients with chronic kidney disease. Ann Intern Med 2010;153:23–33.

100. Jing Z, Wei-jie Y, Nan Z, et al. Hemoglobin targets for chronic kidney disease patients with anemia: a systematic review and meta-analysis. PLoS One 2012;7:e43655.

101. Cleland JG, Daubert JC, Erdmann E, et al, Committee C-H study Steering Investigators. The CARE-HF study (Cardiac Resynchronisation in Heart Failure study): rationale, design and end-points. Eur J Heart Fail 2001;3:481–9.

102. Boerrigter G, Costello-Boerrigter LC, Abraham WT, et al. Cardiac resynchronization therapy improves renal function in human heart failure with reduced glomerular filtration rate. J Card Fail 2008;14:539–46.

103. Bansal N, Tighiouart F, Weiner D, et al. Anemia as a risk factor for kidney function decline in individuals with heart failure. Am J Cardiol 2007;99:1137–42.

104. Spittell PC, Hayes DL. Venous complications after insertion of a transvenous pacemaker. Mayo Clin Proc 1992;67:258–65.

105. Herzog CA, Li S, Weinhandl ED, et al. Survival of dialysis patients after cardiac arrest and the impact of implantable cardioverter defibrillators. Kidney Int 2005;68:818–25.

106. Khan F, Adelstein E, Saba S. Implantable cardioverter defibrillators confer survival benefit in patients with renal insufficiency but not in dialysis-dependent patients. J Interv Card Electrophysiol 2010;28:117–23.

107. Green D, Roberts PR, New DI, et al. Sudden cardiac death in hemodialysis patients: an in-depth review. Am J Kidney Dis 2011;57:921–9.

108. U.S. Renal Data System. USRDS 2013 annual data report: atlas of chronic kidney disease and end-stage renal disease in the United States. 2013. p. 1, 2. Available at: http://www.usrds.org/atlas.aspx.

109. Effect of enalapril on survival in patients with reduced left ventricular ejection fractions and congestive heart failure. The SOLVD investigators. N Engl J Med 1991;325:293–302.

110. McMurray JJ, Ostergren J, Swedberg K, et al, CHARM Investigators and Committees. Effects of candesartan in patients with chronic heart failure and reduced left-ventricular systolic function taking angiotensin-converting-enzyme inhibitors: the CHARM-added trial. Lancet 2003;362:767–71.

111. Cleland JG, Daubert JC, Erdmann E, et al. Cardiac Resynchronization-Heart Failure Study I. The effect of cardiac resynchronization on morbidity and mortality in heart failure. N Engl J Med 2005;352:1539–49.

112. Effects of enalapril on mortality in severe congestive heart failure. Results of the Cooperative North Scandinavian Enalapril Survival Study (Consensus). The Consensus Trial Study Group. N Engl J Med 1987;316:1429–35.

113. Effect of metoprolol CR/XL in chronic heart failure: metoprolol CR/XL randomised intervention trial in congestive heart failure (MERIT-HF). Lancet 1999;353:2001–7.

114. The Cardiac Insufficiency Bisoprolol Study II (CIBIS-II): a randomised trial. Lancet 1999;353:9–13.

115. Packer M, Coats AJ, Fowler MB, et al, Carvedilol Prospective Randomized Cumulative Survival Study Group. Effect of carvedilol on survival in severe chronic heart failure. N Engl J Med 2001;344:1651–8.

116. Dargie HJ. Effect of carvedilol on outcome after myocardial infarction in patients with left-ventricular dysfunction: the Capricorn randomised trial. Lancet 2001;357:1385–90.

117. Digitalis Investigation Group. The effect of digoxin on mortality and morbidity in patients with heart failure. N Engl J Med 1997;336:525–33.

118. Swedberg K, Komajda M, Bohm M, et al, SHIFT Investigators. Ivabradine and outcomes in chronic heart failure (SHIFT): a randomised placebo-controlled study. Lancet 2010;376:875–85.

119. Taylor AL, Ziesche S, Yancy C, et al, African-American Heart Failure Trial Investigators. Combination of isosorbide dinitrate and hydralazine in blacks with heart failure. N Engl J Med 2004;351:2049–57.

120. Moss AJ, Zareba W, Hall WJ, et al, Multicenter Automatic Defibrillator Implantation Trial II Investigators. Prophylactic implantation of a defibrillator in patients with myocardial infarction and reduced ejection fraction. N Engl J Med 2002; 346:877–83.

121. Moss AJ, Hall WJ, Cannom DS, et al. Cardiac-resynchronization therapy for the prevention of heart-failure events. N Engl J Med 2009;361: 1329–38.

Contrast Media
History and Chemical Properties

Michael Buschur, MD[a],*, Peter Aspelin, MD, PhD[b]

KEYWORDS

- Contrast media • Cardiac catheterization • History

KEY POINTS

- Contrast media, which are essential for cardiac catheterization, are classified based on water solubility and osmolality.
- Contrast media were discovered during the search for a treatment of syphilis, and initial agents were developed in urology.
- Contrast media agents have evolved from high-osmolar agents with many side effects to low-osmolar and iso-osmolar agents with considerably fewer side effects to the patient.

INTRODUCTION

Since the time of Hippocrates, physicians have sought better tools to diagnose disease. Röntgen's discovery of x-rays enabled physicians to use this modality in improving diagnosis of disease in patients. Radiology has rapidly evolved, and the improvement has partly been successful thanks to different types of contrast media that have been invented to better visualize tissues.

Cardiac catheterization uses x-rays and contrast agents to visualize the heart. Contrast agents are essential for imaging the cardiac chambers and coronary vessels, and the evolution of contrast agents has had a significant effect on cardiology.

This article reviews the classification of contrast agents, a brief history of development of contrast agents, and the chemical properties of agents currently used in cardiac catheterization.

CLASSIFICATION OF CONTRAST AGENTS

All contrast media used in cardiology are distributed intravascularly and extracellularly. They are classified into ionic and nonionic groups based on water solubility. Ionic agents are water soluble, as they dissociate into negative and positive ions. These ions then bind with the negative and positive poles of water molecules. Nonionic agents do not dissociate but are water soluble because of their polar OH groups.[1]

Contrast agents are further divided based on their osmolality into high-osmolar contrast media (HOCM), low-osmolar contrast media (LOCM), and iso-osmolar contrast media (IOCM). **Box 1** lists some of the most common contrast agents sorted by class. Contrast agent ratio is used to further classify contrast media; this ratio is calculated by the number of iodine atoms divided by the number of particles in solution. **Table 1** shows the differences in osmolality and contrast agent ratios for some contrast media. Iodine content in relation to osmotic particles per molecule is the most important factor impacting attenuation.[1,2]

All contrast agents have a basic structure of a benzene ring, which is composed of 6 joined carbon atoms, each of which has an attached

The authors have nothing to disclose.
[a] Division of Cardiovascular Medicine, University of Michigan, 1500 East Medical Center Drive, Ann Arbor, MI 48109, USA; [b] Division of Medical Imaging and Technology, Department of Clinical Science, Intervention and Technology, Karolinska University Hospital, Karolinska Institutet, Stockholm, SE 14186, Sweden
* Corresponding author.
E-mail address: mbuschur@med.umich.edu

Intervent Cardiol Clin 3 (2014) 333–339
http://dx.doi.org/10.1016/j.iccl.2014.03.008

Box 1
Classification of contrast media

Ionic media
- Monomers: high-osmolar contrast media
  - Examples: ioxithalamic acids, diatrizoate
- Dimers: low-osmolar contrast media
  - Example: ioxaglate

Nonionic media
- Monomers: low-osmolar contrast media
  - Examples: iohexol, iopamidol, ioversol, iopromide
- Dimers: iso-osmolar contrast media
  - Examples: iodixanol, iotrolan

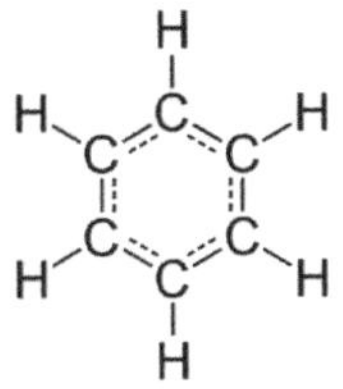

Fig. 1. A benzene ring is composed of 6 joined carbon atoms, each of which has an attached hydrogen atom. Dashed lines represent delocalization of electrons over the carbon atoms. C, carbon atom; H, hydrogen atom.

hydrogen atom (**Fig. 1**). Contrast media consist of triiodinated benzene rings, whereby 3 hydrogen atoms are replaced with attached iodine atoms. Monomers contain 1 triiodinated benzene ring, and dimers contain 2 triiodinated benzene rings. Attachment at the first carbon atom differentiates ionic from nonionic contrast agents, with sodium or another cation, such as meglumine, attached in ionic agents and an amide group attached in nonionic agents. The iodine molecule is attached at carbon atoms 2, 4, and 6. Iodine has a tight bond to the carbon atoms, which augments attenuation by increasing the linear coefficient of radiation. Side chains containing OH groups are attached at carbon atoms 1, 3, and 5 and functions to raise solubility and decrease protein binding.

HISTORY OF IMAGING

In 1895, at The University of Wurzburg, Wilhelm Conrad Röntgen discovered x-ray by passing electrical charges through vacuum tubes. The letter x was used, as it was the mathematical term to designate an unknown variable.[3] Within a month after Röntgen's discovery, x-rays began to be used for medical purposes.[4] However, initial x-rays were low power and made visualization difficult. By 1896, more than 1000 papers had been published on x-rays, including 500 publications on x-rays used for medical applications.[5]

X-rays were quickly found to have limitations and required enhancement to produce better images. Haschek and Lindenthal in Vienna discovered that bismuth, lead, and elements with high atomic numbers enhanced x-ray images but were not safe for use in humans.[6] Therefore, the search for optimal, safe contrast agents continued.

Advancements in imaging were first made in imaging of the urinary tract. In 1897, Hurry Fenwick used x-rays to detect kidney stones before urologic surgery.[7,8] He then introduced bougies infused with metal into the ureters, enabling the visualization of the course of the ureters and localization of calculi with x-ray imaging.[4]

To further improve visualization with x-rays, a radiopaque agent administration was necessary. In 1906, Von Lichtenberg and Voelcker used an agent to create retrograde pyelographic studies.[9] They initially used a 2% colloidal silver solution. However, this was found to be toxic to the kidneys, at times even resulting in death.

Table 1
Iodinated contrast media

Classification	Iodine Atoms per Molecule	Osmotic Particles per Molecule	Contrast Agent Ratio	Molecular Weight	Osmolality (Osm/kg Water)
Ionic monomer	3	2	1.5	600–800	1.5–1.7
Nonionic monomer	3	1	3	600–800	0.6–0.7
Ionic dimer	6	2	3	1269	0.56
Nonionic dimer	6	1	6	1550–1626	0.3

Data from Aspelin P, Bellin MF, Jacobsen JA, et al. Classification and terminology. In: Thomsen HS, editor. Contrast media - safety issues and ESUR guidelines. 2nd edition. New York: Springer; 2009. p. 1–4; and Dawson P, Cosgrove DO, Grainger RG, editors. Textbook of contrast media. Oxford (United Kingdom): Isis Medical Media Ltd; 1999.

DEVELOPMENT OF IODINE-BASED CONTRAST MEDIA

During the 1920s at the Mayo Clinic, Osborne and colleagues[10] used a 10% sodium iodide solution for the treatment of syphilis. They fortuitously discovered that sodium iodide was radiopaque and excreted by the kidneys and then performed the first pyelogram.

Continuing with using iodine for syphilis treatment, a German team of Arthur Binz and Curt Rath developed many iodine preparations for treatment of the infection. One compound called Selectan was based on the iodination of the pyridine ring, which is composed of 5 carbon atoms and 1 nitrogen atom. Detoxified arsenic and iodine compounds were linked to this ring.[11]

Selectan was then tested in Lichtwitz's laboratory on humans. Moses Swick,[12] a research fellow in the laboratory, determined that Selectan was effective for treatment of urinary tract infections and was rapidly and almost exclusively eliminated by the kidneys. By applying ureteral compression, he discovered that the kidneys and ureters were visible on radiograph, proving Selectan to be a renal contrast medium. Swick then performed experiments with Von Lichtenberg in Berlin, and they completed the first successful intravenous (IV) urogram.

In 1927, Binz and Rath expanded on Selectan by developing new agents for IV urograms.[13] They developed Uroselectan, the sodium salt of 5-iodo-2-pyridone-N-acetic acid, which had increased solubility and less toxicity compared with Selectan. Sodium o-iodohippurate (Hippuran) was introduced by Mallinckrodt Chemical Works in 1933 with cooperation of Swick.[14] The class of Selectans in contrast media was named for their selective excretion by the liver and kidneys.

Binz and Rath continued to develop new compounds based on modifications of the pyridine ring, including neo-ipax (Iodoxyl) and diodrast (Diodone), which were successful commercial products from the Schering-Kahlbaum Company and were the universal agents used for the next 20 years (**Fig. 2**).[2]

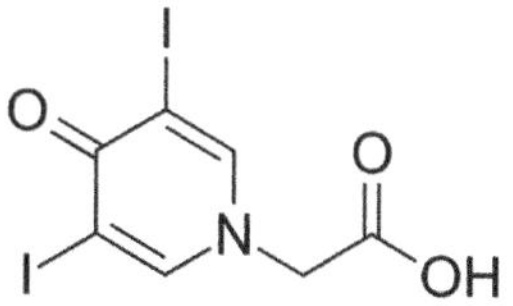

Fig. 2. Chemical structure of diodrast, an ionic monomer (high-osmolar contrast agent media). I, iodine atom; N, nitrogen atom; O, oxygen atom; OH, hydroxyl group. Double line indicates double bond.

BEGINNINGS OF ANGIOGRAPHY

In the late 1920s, Werner Forssmann experimented with cardiac catheterization via self-catheterization. He introduced a urinary catheter in his antecubital vein and advanced the catheter to the right heart. In later experiments, he administered sodium iodide to image his own cardiac chambers. He later used Uroselectan, but was unable to view the right atrium and reported feeling faint and developed a warm sensation in his mouth.[15,16]

In 1923, Berberich and Hirsch performed the first femoral angiogram. Soon after, in 1924, Brooks used sodium iodide to perform the first angiogram.[17] He performed angiograms of the lower extremities in patients with ulcers and gangrene to visualize the vascular system to help surgeons assess where to amputate. Patients required general anesthesia for performance of angiograms as they experienced severe pain with the injection of sodium iodide.

In 1926, Moniz performed a cerebral arteriogram, which is one of the most famous achievements in angiography. He injected 5 mL of a 25% aqueous solution of sodium iodide directly into the internal carotid artery to visualize the cerebral vasculature.[18]

DEVELOPMENT OF HOCM

High-osmolar contrast agents (HOCM) are agents with a single, negatively charged triiodinated benzene ring attached to sodium or another cation, such as meglumine. The benzene ring has 3 hydrogen atoms replaced by iodine atoms and 3 hydrogen atoms replaced by simple side chains. Only the negatively charged anion is radiopaque.[19] The sodium content of the agents is equivalent to that of blood. HOCM are monomers that dissociate and ionize in solution with a valence of -1. Although they are the oldest contrast agents and are inexpensive, their utility is limited because of cardiotoxicity related to calcium binding and repolarization charges.

Vernon Wallingford,[20] a research chemist at Mallinckrodt Chemical Works, experimented by making substantial changes to the pyridine ring, resulting in new, safer contrast agents. Working with Moses Swick, Wallingford introduced a 6-carbon benzene ring as the iodine carrier compared with the 5-carbon and 1-nitrogen ring previously used by Binz and Rath. He expanded on the benzene ring by adding an acetyl-amino group, creating the first triiodinated contrast medium, which was called sodium acetrizoate (Urokon) in 1951 (**Fig. 3**). Urokon was the sodium salt of

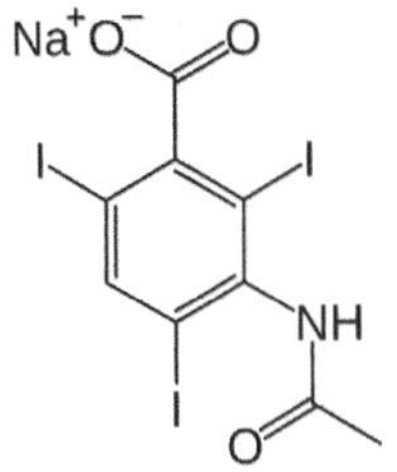

Fig. 3. Chemical structure of sodium acetrizoate, an ionic monomer (high-osmolar contrast media). I, iodine atom; Na, sodium atom; NH, amine group; O, oxygen atom. Double line indicates double bond.

3-acetylamin-2,4,6 triiodobenzoic acid, which was 10 times as soluble and one-sixth as toxic as previous compounds.[21] Around the same time, Swick discovered that Uroselectan amplified x-ray contrast after IV injection.

Wallingford developed similar media (Miokon among others) based on Urokon, all of which are the triiodinated benzoic acid and contain acylamino groups. Initially, these were developed for urography but were quickly expanded to other fields of medicine.[20]

In 1956, Hoppe created sodium diatrizoate by adding a second acetyl-amino group to the benzene ring (**Fig. 4**). Animal studies showed this agent had reduced toxicity, and it was then marketed as Hypaque.[22] Hypaque and its derivatives were the standard contrast agents used until the 1970s. Hypaque and similar agents are ionic monomer salts, containing 3 iodine atoms and 1 cation. The cation is necessary to produce the salt molecule and consists of sodium, N-methylglucamine (meglumine), or a mixture of the 2 salts.

In regard to coronary angiography, a mixture of the sodium and meglumine salts is necessary to reduce cardiac toxicity and arrhythmias as described by Gensini and Di Giorgi.[23] This combination of the 2 cations led to the development of Isopaque and its variations, which are composed of various combinations of sodium, meglumine, magnesium, and calcium.

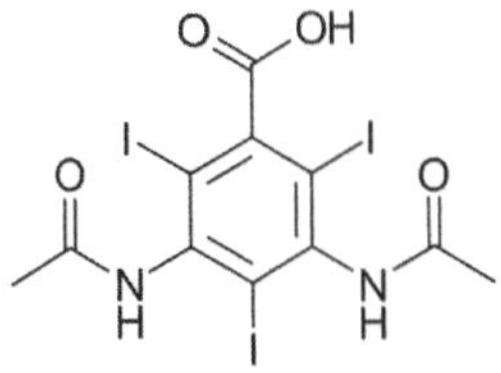

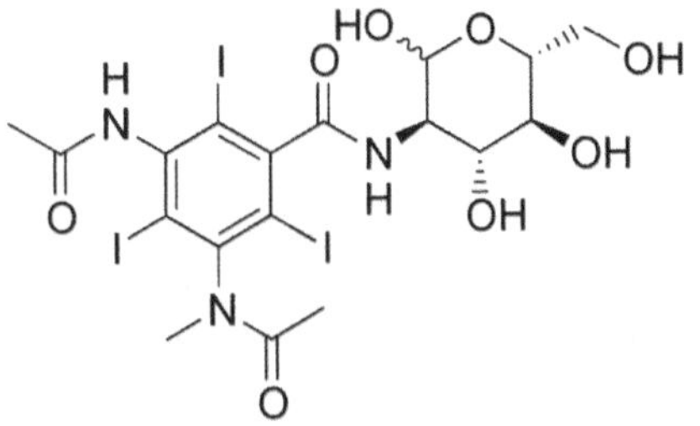

Fig. 5. Chemical structure of metrizamide, a nonionic monomer (low-osmolar contrast media). Double line indicates double bond. Dashed line indicates single bond with stereochemistry pointing into the page. Wedge line indicates single bond with stereochemistry pointing out of the page. Squiggly line indicates unknown stereochemistry. I, iodine atom; N, nitrogen atom; NH, amine group; O, oxygen atom; OH, hydroxyl group.

Although the HOCM agents furthered radiographic visualization and represented great advancements, they continued to have significant side effects because of their osmolality, which was 5 to 8 times the physiologic concentration. These agents adversely affect erythrocytes, permeability of capillary endothelium, and circulating blood volume.[24] Side effects ranged from minor reactions such as flushing and nausea to more severe reactions including bronchospasm, pulmonary edema, contrast-induced nephropathy, and even death.[25] Owing to the severity of side effects, better agents were clearly needed.

DEVELOPMENT OF CONTRAST MEDIA WITH A BETTER SAFETY PROFILE

Torsten Almén,[26] a Swedish radiologist, noted that the pain with angiography was associated with the osmolality. He thus proclaimed that osmolality was

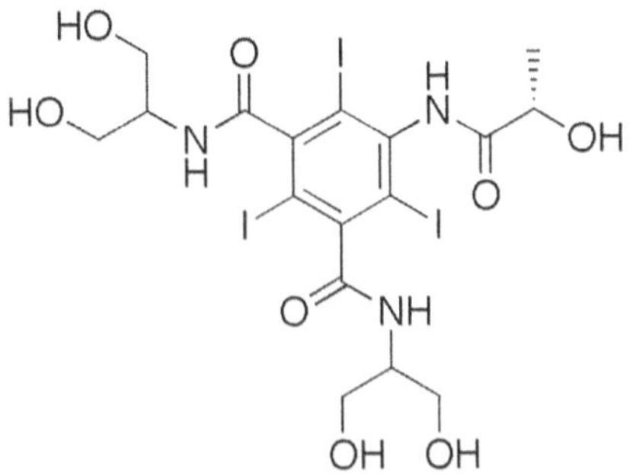

Fig. 6. Chemical structure of iopamidol, a nonionic monomer (low-osmolar contrast media). I, iodine atom; NH, amine group; O, oxygen atom; OH, hydroxyl group. Dashed line indicates single bond with stereochemistry pointing into the page. Double line indicates double bond.

Fig. 4. Chemical structure of sodium diatrizoate, an ionic monomer (high-osmolar contrast media). I, iodine atom; NH, amine group; O, oxygen atom; OH, hydroxyl group. Double line indicates double bond.

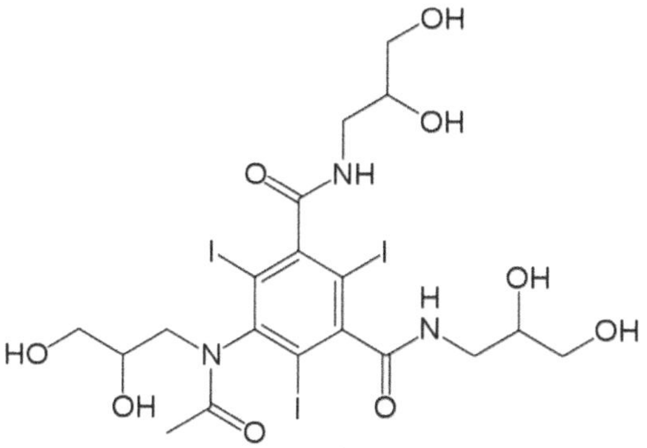

Fig. 7. Chemical structure of iohexol, a nonionic monomer (low-osmolar contrast media). I, iodine atom; N, nitrogen atom; NH, amine group; O, oxygen atom; OH, hydroxyl group. Double line indicates double bond.

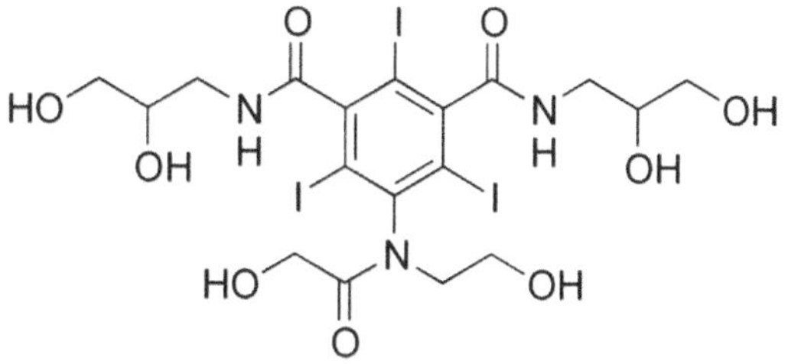

Fig. 9. Chemical structure of ioversol, a nonionic monomer (low-osmolar contrast media). I, iodine atom; N, nitrogen atom; NH, amine group; O, oxygen atom; OH, hydroxyl group. Double line indicates double bond.

responsible for much of the contrast media toxicity. He therefore suggested that one should develop contrast media with reduced osmolality. He suggested the substitution of the cation with a radical to an amide, as well as the creation of dimers. The major radiological journals did not accept his suggestion, but it was published in 1969 in the *Journal of Theoretical Biology*.

DEVELOPMENT OF LOCM

Torsten Almén, after his suggestions of reducing osmolality, worked with the pharmaceutical company Nyegaard, and they produced metrizamide (Amipaque), the first LOCM in 1969 and introduced it in 1972 (**Fig. 5**). This agent had excellent results with no pain in 20 patients undergoing femoral angiography.[27] Metrizamide is a combination of metrizoic acid and glucosamine, which was water soluble with low osmolality. The osmolality was 485 mOsm, and the vascular pain threshold is between 600 and 700 mOsm. The use of this agent was unfortunately limited, as it precipitates at

high temperatures such are necessary with sterilization.[6]

A major advance was therefore the further development of these nonionic compounds, which are monomers that dissolve in water but do not dissociate. Therefore, nonionic compounds have fewer particles in solution and are designated LOCM. Nonionic agents minimize side effects related to hypertonicity. Examples of nonionic agents include iopamidol (Iopamiro), iohexol (Omnipaque), iopromide (Ultravist), ioversol (Optiray), and iobitridol (Xenetix) (**Figs. 6–10**).

In the 1970s, the French company Guerbet and the British company Baker together developed a new medium called ioxaglate (Hexabrix) by combining 2 triiodinated benzene rings (**Fig. 11**). Benzene rings have a carboxylic acid group. When the 2 rings are combined, 1 ring has its carboxylic acid group converted to a nonionizing radical and the other benzene ring has its carboxylic acid group converted to an ionizing salt such as sodium or meglumine. Hexabrix is an ionic contrast agent, but it has an iodine atom to particle ratio of 6:2, which is equivalent to the 3:1 ratio of the other low-osmolar media such as iohexol and iopamidol.[28] However, although Hexabrix was an

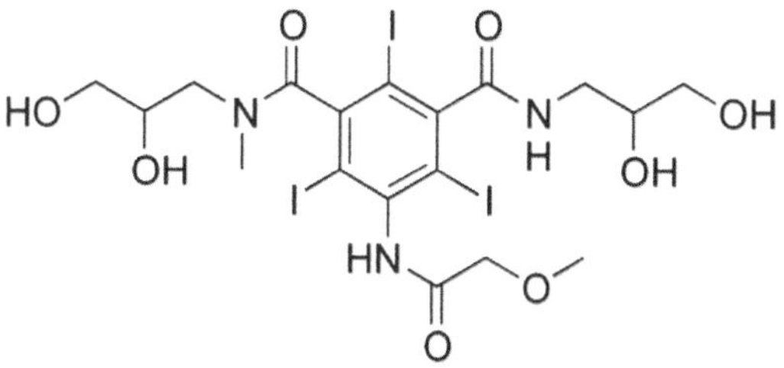

Fig. 8. Chemical structure of iopromide, a nonionic monomer (low-osmolar contrast media). I, iodine atom; N, nitrogen atom; NH, amine group; O, oxygen atom; OH, hydroxyl group. Double line indicates double bond.

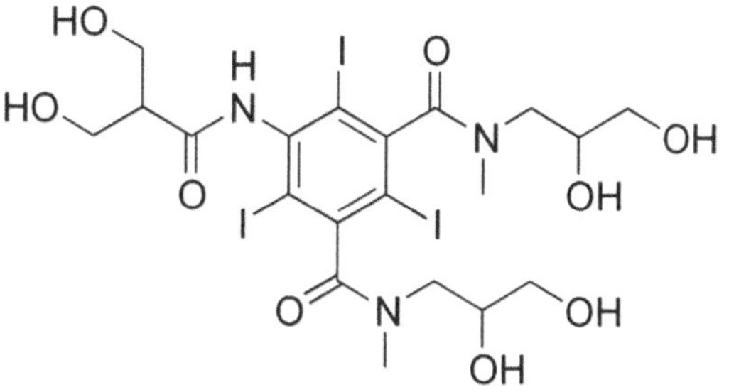

Fig. 10. Chemical structure of iobitridol, a nonionic monomer (low-osmolar contrast media). I, iodine atom; N, nitrogen atom; NH, amine group; O, oxygen atom; OH, hydroxyl group. Double line indicates double bond.

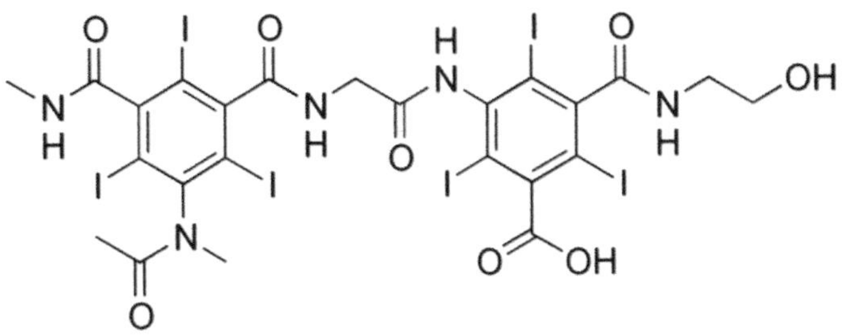

Fig. 11. Chemical structure of ioxaglate, an ionic dimer (low-osmolar contrast media). I, iodine atom; N, nitrogen atom; NH, amine group; O, oxygen atom; OH, hydroxyl group. Double line indicates double bond.

effective arterial agent, its use was limited because of severe nausea and vomiting on IV injection. Hexabrix resulted in significantly less pain and less hypotension than sodium diatrizoate, with no difference in radiographic properties.[29] Furthermore, the LOCM agents resulted in less cardiac depression during angiography, blood volume increases, renal toxicity, and anaphylactic reactions.[13,30]

During the next 10 years, advances were made to these agents, making them more stable, easier to manufacture, and cheaper. These LOCM agents remain the intravascular agents of choice today. These agents have many advantages over older agents, including the following: lack of a glucose radical, ability to be autoclaved, easier synthesis, and less expensive to produce. Simple sugar moieties were replaced with hydrophilic, water-soluble sugar moieties, which made these agents better than metrizamide with retained high osmolality.

DEVELOPMENT OF IOCM

The most recent class of contrast agents consist of a molecule with 2 benzene rings (each with 3 iodine atoms) that are nonionic and thus do not dissociate in water. These compounds are classified as IOCM. The toxicity of contrast agents decreases as their osmolality approaches that of serum. Reducing osmolality in nonionizing compounds has been accomplished by joining 2 monomers to create a dimer. Iodixanol (Visipaque) is the only IOCM used in the cardiac catheterization laboratory (Fig. 12).

VISCOSITY

Although viscosity is not as important as osmolality, contrast agents should still have the lowest attainable viscosity. Although experimental studies in rats have shown that contrast media may induce high viscosity in the renal tubules, affecting renal function, this has not been confirmed in human studies. Instead, contrast media with the lowest viscosity (high-osmolar contrast agents) are much more nephrotoxic than those with higher viscosity (low- and iso-osmolar contrast agents).

The main factors affecting viscosity are the iodine concentration, the temperature, and the size of the molecule. Therefore, dimers have higher viscosity than monomers and the ionic contrast media have a lower viscosity than the nonionic.

In cardiac angiography today, however, viscosity is of minor importance because heating of the contrast media and autoinjectors reduce most of the problems that a high-viscosity agent may have.

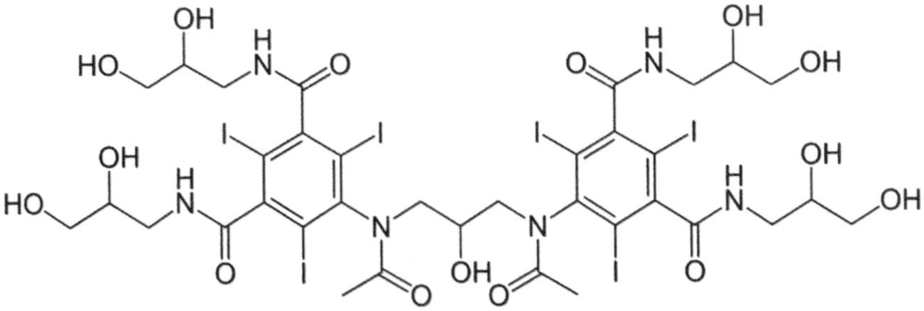

Fig. 12. Chemical structure of iodixanol, a nonionic dimer (iso-osmolar contrast media). I, iodine atom; N, nitrogen atom; NH, amine group; O, oxygen atom; OH, hydroxyl group. Double line indicates double bond.

SUMMARY

Despite the tremendous advancements in contrast media since the discovery of x-ray technology, continued research is needed for agents that can achieve high concentration in body tissues with less toxicity. From a contrast standpoint, Uroselectan was a turning point, which led to marked research and development in contrast media. With the advancement of LOCM and IOCM, toxicity continues to be reduced with maintenance of high-quality imaging for advancement of patient care.

REFERENCES

1. Aspelin P, Bellin MF, Jacobsen JA, et al. Contrast media - safety issues and ESUR guidelines. Classification and terminology. 2nd edition. Germany: Springer Verlag; 2009.
2. Dawson P, Cosgrove DO, Grainger RG, editors. Textbook of contrast media. Oxford (United Kingdom): Isis Medical Media Ltd; 1999.
3. Grigg E. The trail of the invisible light from X-Strahlen to Radio(bio)logy. In: Thomas C, editor. Springfield; 1965.
4. Rigler LG. Roentgen diagnosis of the upper gastrointestinal tract. Historical development. J Lancet 1962;82:293–300.
5. Spiegel P. The first clinical X-ray made in America– 100 years. Am J Roentgenol 1995;164(1):241–3.
6. Quader MA, Sawmiller CJ, Sumpio BA. Radio Contrast Agents: History and Evolution. In: Chang JB, Olsen ER, Prasad K, et al. Textbook of Angiology. New York: Springer; 2000. p. 775–83.
7. Fenwick EH. The Roentgen rays and the fluoroscope as a means of detecting small, deeply placed stones in the exposed kidney. Br Med J 1897; 2(1920):1075–7.
8. Fenwick EH. An operative demonstration of the occasional diagnostic accuracy of the X-ray in urinary stone. Br Med J 1908;1(2453):4–1.b3.
9. Eisendrath D, Rolnick HC. Urology. 4th edition. Philadelphia: JB Lippincott Company; 1938.
10. Osborne ED, Sutherland CG, Scholl AJ Jr, et al. Landmark article Feb 10, 1923: Roentgenography of urinary tract during excretion of sodium iodide. By Earl D. Osborne, Charles G. Sutherland, Albert J. Scholl, Jr. and Leonard G. Rowntree. JAMA 1983;250(20):2848–53.
11. Binz A, Rath C. Uber biochemische Eigenschaften von Derivaten des Pyridines und Chinolins. Biochem Z 1928;203:218–22.
12. Swick M. Darstellung der Niere und Harnwege im Roentgenbild durch untravenose Einbringung eines neuen Kontrastsoffes, des Uroselectans. Verhandl d deutsch Gesellsch f Urol, IX Kongress, Munich 1929;9:328–31.
13. Rapoport S, Bookstein JJ, Higgins CB, et al. Experience with metrizamide in patients with previous severe anaphylactoid reactions to ionic contrast agents. Radiology 1982;143(2):321–5.
14. Swick M. Intravenous urography by means of the sodium salt of 5-iodo-2-pyridon-N-acetic acid. From the Journal of the American Medical Association, Nov. 8, 1930, Vol. 95, pp. 1403–1409. Mt Sinai J Med 2003;70(4):269–79.
15. Hricak H, Barbariv ZL. Newer imaging techniques: workshop. In: Robinson I, editor. Proc 9th Int Congr Nephrol, Los Angeles; 1984. p. 1430–6.
16. Forsmann W. The catheterization of the right side of the heart. Klin Wochenschr 1929;8:2085–7.
17. Brooks B. Intra-arterial injection of sodium iodide. JAMA 1924;82(13):1016–9.
18. Brewer AJ, editor. Classic descriptions in diagnostic roentgenology. Springfield (IL): Thomas; 1964.
19. Grainger R. Future prospects in diagnostic radiology. Proc R Soc Med 1971;64:243–9.
20. Wallingford VH. General aspects of contrast media research. Ann N Y Acad Sci 1959;78:707–19.
21. Wallingford V, Decker HG, Kruty M. X-ray contrast media. Iodinated acylaminobenzoic acids. J Am Chem Soc 1952;74:4365.
22. Hoppe JO, Larsen AA, Coulston F. Observations on the toxicity of a new urographic contrast medium, sodium 3, 5-diacetamido-2, 4, 6-triiodobenzoate (hypaquesodium) and related compounds. J Pharmacol Exp Ther 1956;116(4):394–403.
23. Gensini G, Di Giorgi S. Myocardial Toxicity of Contrast Agents Used in Angiography. Radiology 1964;82:24–34.
24. Grainger RG. Osmolality of intravascular radiological contrast media. Br J Radiol 1980;53(632):739–46.
25. Ansell G, Tweedie MC, West CR, et al. The current status of reactions to intravenous contrast media. Invest Radiol 1980;15(Suppl 6):S32–9.
26. Almén T. Contrast agent design. Some aspects on the synthesis of water-soluble contrast agents of low osmolality. J Theor Biol 1969;24:216–26.
27. Almen T, Boijsen E, Lindell SE. Metrizamide in angiography I. Femoral angiography. Acta Radiol Diagn (Stockh) 1977;18(1):33–8.
28. Dawson P, Grainger RG, Pitfield J. The new low-osmolar contrast media: a simple guide. Clin Radiol 1983;34(2):221–6.
29. Holm M, Praestholm J. Ioxaglate, a new low osmolar contrast medium used in femoral angiography. Br J Radiol 1979;52(615):169–72.
30. Higgins CB. Effects of contrast materials on left ventricular function. Invest Radiol 1980;15(Suppl 6): S220–31.

Nonrenal Complications of Contrast Media

 CrossMark

Damien Marycz, MD, Khaled M. Ziada, MD*

KEYWORDS

- Contrast media • Anaphylactoid reactions • Preoperative treatment • Chemotoxicity

KEY POINTS

- Chemotoxic reactions to contrast media are mostly related to ionicity and osmolality; these have become less significant with the nonionic iso-osmolar agents more commonly used today.
- Anaphylactoid reactions to contrast media are secondary to release of histamine and other vasoactive substances, but cannot be considered typical of true anaphylactic reactions, which are mediated by immunoglobulin E antibodies.
- Patients who have had a previous anaphylactoid reaction to contrast or those with atopic conditions are at increased risk for adverse reactions to contrast, and should be targeted for preventive treatment before repeat exposure.
- A history of seafood or shellfish allergy is not associated with an increased risk for anaphylactoid reactions to contrast media.
- Appropriate medical pretreatment to avoid anaphylactoid reactions must include prednisone, with at least 1 dose administered more than 12 hours before contrast injection.
- Patients undergoing immunotherapy treatment with recombinant interleukin 2 have been shown to have an increased risk for the development of delayed adverse reactions to contrast media.

Injection of contrast media is the foundation of invasive and interventional cardiovascular practice. Iodine-based contrast was first safely used in the 1920s for urologic procedures and examinations. Initially these agents were poorly tolerated owing to the side effects of nausea, vomiting, and hypotension related to the very high ionic and osmolar concentrations. In the 1950s, the triiodobenzoic acid derivatives were developed (sodium and meglumine salts of triiodinated benzoic acid derivatives), which contained lower ionic concentrations and had lower osmolarity than the contrast agents originally used. These newer agents, with their lower ionic and osmolar concentration, were more hydrophilic and better tolerated by patients because of their less chemotoxic profiles.[1]

Despite the high safety profile of iodinated contrast agents, their use can be associated with side effects and complications. Contrast-induced nephropathy is one of the major concerns associated with the use of these agents in the catheterization laboratory and radiology suites (see later discussion). This article is dedicated to the discussion of all nonrenal side effects and complications related to the use of contrast agents in the catheterization laboratory.

There are 2 major classes of side effects and complications related to contrast media: chemotoxicity and anaphylactoid reactions. Chemotoxicity is related to the physical and chemical properties of the agent used, whereas anaphylactoid reactions are probably related to the iodine content

The authors have nothing to disclose.
Division of Cardiovascular Medicine, Gill Heart Institute, University of Kentucky, 900 South Limestone Street, 326 Wethington Building, Lexington, KY 40536-0200, USA
* Corresponding author.
E-mail address: khaled.ziada@uky.edu

interventional.theclinics.com

(**Fig. 1**). The various reactions, their clinical presentations, and management strategies are discussed in detail.

CHEMOTOXIC REACTIONS

Chemotoxic reactions are related to the chemical properties, dose, and rate of infusion of the contrast agent used. The typical minor chemotoxic reactions of contrast media include nausea, flushing, warmth, and pain at the injection site. The major chemotoxic reactions include hypotension, dysrhythmias, depressed myocardial contractility, and myocardial ischemia. The ionic concentration, osmolality, viscosity, and calcium-binding properties of these contrast agents are responsible for most types of reactions.

These reactions were more frequent and more severe in the earlier days of angiography, when contrast media were ionic and had high osmolality (up to1400 mOsm/kg). As significant volumes of such agents are injected in the intravascular space, a dramatic increase in intravascular osmolality ensues, which in turn leads to fluid shift from the intracellular to the extracellular spaces. The intravascular volume increase manifests as an elevation of the left ventricular end-diastolic pressure, pulmonary edema, and cellular dysfunction.[2] Electrophysiologic effects of ionic contrast media included decreased rate of depolarization of the sinoatrial node, PR-interval prolongation, and, occasionally, heart block or even ventricular fibrillation. The electrophysiologic effects are thought to be caused by transient hypocalcemia via binding of calcium from the radiopaque anion in addition to calcium-sequestering agents (such as sodium citrate and sodium ethylenediaminetetraacetic acid) often used in ionic contrast agents of high osmolarity.[3,4] The use of ionic high-osmolar contrast agents was also known to produce a transient depression in myocardial performance and was responsible for the hypotension seen with the use of these agents. This decrease in blood pressure can further lead to myocardial ischemia and circulatory collapse in patients with severe coronary ischemia, decompensated heart failure, or critical aortic stenosis.

Modifications to the ionic structure and iodine content of contrast media in the 1980s led to the development of ionic low-osmolar contrast media, nonionic low-osmolar contrast media, and nonionic iso-osmolar contrast media. By virtue of their lower osmolality and low ionic concentrations, these contrast agents are better tolerated by patients and produce fewer major side effects in comparison with ionic high-osmolar contrast agents.

ACUTE AND EARLY ANAPHYLACTOID REACTIONS

Anaphylactoid reactions to contrast media are typically divided into 2 classes related to the onset of the reaction in relation to the time of contrast exposure: acute or early reactions occur within 1 hour of delivery, and delayed reactions occur within 1 hour to 7 days after exposure (see **Fig. 1**).[5]

Manifestations and Incidence

The acute reactions are typically characterized as being allergic-like reactions or physiologic reactions to the chemical properties of the contrast media. The severity of these reactions can range

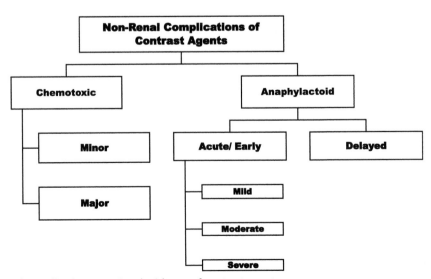

Fig. 1. Types of complications associated with use of contrast agents.

from minor cutaneous reactions (such as rash or urticaria) to severe life-threatening reactions such as circulatory collapse and shock (**Table 1**). Observational studies from the 1980s showed that mild acute reactions occurred in 3.8% to 12.7% of patients receiving ionic, high-osmolar contrast and in 0.7% to 3.1% of patients receiving lower-osmolar nonionic contrast. The frequency of immediate severe acute reactions has been reported to be 0.1% to 0.4% for ionic contrast and 0.02% to 0.04% for nonionic contrast media.[6–9]

Pathophysiology

The exact pathophysiology causing these reactions is not completely understood and does not seem to result from an observable antigen-antibody interaction. Hence these reactions are referred to as anaphylactoid, idiosyncratic, allergic-like, or pseudoallergic reactions.[10] Most of these reactions are thought to be related to the release of histamine from basophils and mast cells in addition to other vasoactive substances, or by direct activation of the complement system.[6] In rare cases, immunoglobulin E (IgE) antibodies (which are the hallmark of true anaphylaxis) have been reported in the literature as another potential mechanism in the hypersensitivity reactions associated with certain iodinated contrast media.[11,12]

Laboratory Testing

Although not frequently used in clinical practice, blood tests can confirm the diagnosis at the time of the acute anaphylactoid reaction. Serum levels of histamine may be elevated in some, but not all individuals after an acute severe anaphylactoid reaction.[13] Tryptase levels have also been found to be elevated in this setting; blood analysis may be obtained at the time of symptom onset and several days after resolution for comparison.[14]

Skin testing by skin prick, intradermal, and patch methods can be used to identify patients at risk for reactions, particularly those who have reported a prior anaphylactoid reaction and are expected to require a repeat exposure to contrast. Several studies using skin testing have confirmed that the cause of acute severe reactions to contrast is immune mediated (and possibly mediated by IgE) and can aid in determining a contrast medium that is less likely to cause a severe reaction in those with a prior history.[15–17] These skin tests should be conducted with caution, as there is some concern for developing an acute severe allergic reaction to the test itself.

TREATMENT OF ACUTE ANAPHYLACTOID REACTIONS

Intermediate-type reactions can be more serious and are usually quick to respond to appropriate therapy. These intermediate reactions include diffuse erythema or urticaria, hoarseness, mild dyspnea and bronchospasm, or transient hypotension. Although these types of reactions are usually quick to respond to treatment, if not done in a timely fashion they may lead to more severe life-threatening reactions.

Severe reactions to contrast media that are life-threatening include seizures, angioedema, laryngeal edema, or severe bronchospasm causing airway compromise, pulmonary edema, arrhythmias, and circulatory collapse.[18]

It is critically important to distinguish between vasovagal reactions and anaphylactoid reactions. Both can result in flushing, nausea, vomiting, and/or hypotension, which can be profound. Vasodepressor reactions differ in that they are associated with bradycardia and heart rate usually of less than 50 beats per minute, whereas hypotension of severe anaphylactoid reactions is commonly associated with tachycardia. The exact cause of vasovagal reactions to contrast media is not clearly identified, but may be related to chemical properties of the contrast agent on the central nervous system. These reactions may also be related to anxiety associated with the procedure, placing an intravenous needle, or the sight of one's own blood.[19] Differentiation of vasovagal reactions from anaphylactoid reactions is crucial, as treatment options are significantly different.

For mild reactions, patients should be observed after the procedure and discharged only once their symptoms have been resolved (**Table 2**). Frequently the symptoms resolve spontaneously, and no additional therapy is needed. In some cases, intravenous ondansetron (4 mg) or prochlorperazine (12.5 mg) can be used to treat

Table 1 Classification of anaphylactoid reactions		
Minor	**Moderate**	**Severe**
Nausea	Mild dyspnea	Angioedema
Vomiting	Bronchospasm	Laryngeal edema
Flushing	Transient hypotension	Cardiovascular shock
Limited urticaria	Diffuse urticaria	Ventricular tachycardia
Erythema	Diffuse erythema	Cardiorespiratory arrest
		Seizures

Table 2
Commonly used therapeutic agents for the treatment of chemotoxic and anaphylactoid contrast reactions

Reaction	Medication(s)	Dose	Comments
Nausea	Ondansetron	4 mg intravenously over 2–5 min	Can cause QT prolongation
	Prochlorperazine	2.5–12.5 mg intravenously	
Urticaria	Diphenhydramine	25–50 mg oral or intravenously	Central nervous system depression is common
Bronchospasm (mild)	β2 Agonist	Albuterol, 2 puffs (90 μg/puff, for a total of 180 μg)	Common side effects include palpations, tremor, and tachycardia
	Supplemental oxygen	By nasal cannula or face mask	Maintain oximetry >92%
Bronchospasm (moderate to severe)	Epinephrine	1:1000 dilution, 0.1–0.3 mg (0.1–0.3 mL) subcutaneously or 1:10,000 dilution, 0.1–0.3 mg (1–3 mL) intravenously	Monitor closely for tachycardia or other arrhythmias
	β2 Agonist	Albuterol sulfate inhalation, 0.83% Nebulized solution, 2.5–5 mg once	Can repeat inhalation of 2.5 mg every 20 min; may cause tachycardia
	Supplemental oxygen	By face mask, 6–10 L/min	Monitor arterial oxygen, arterial blood gas saturation
Laryngeal edema	Epinephrine and β2 agonists	Dosage as outlined above	
	Corticosteroids Methylprednisolone Hydrocortisone	Methylprednisolone, 40 mg intravenously Hydrocortisone, 100–200 mg intravenously	High-dose corticosteroids should generally not be used for >72 h
Symptomatic bradycardia (with or without hypotension)	Atropine	0.5–1 mg intravenously Repeat 0.8–1 mg every 3–5 min	Maximum dose should not exceed a total of 3 mg

persistent nausea and vomiting. Diphenhydramine, 25 to 50 mg intravenously is often adequate to control pruritus associated with mild rash. Clinical judgment is needed to determine whether symptoms will progress and if more aggressive treatment is needed.

For intermediate reactions, patients require longer observation after the procedure and frequent checks on vital signs. In addition to symptomatic treatment of nausea and pruritus, intravenous fluids should be started if there is evidence of hypotension, and intravenous corticosteroids can be considered for diffuse erythema and urticarial reactions.

For severe reactions it is important to recognize the problem immediately, as these are life-threatening situations. The initial management of severe acute reactions begins with assessing airway, breathing, and circulation. Oxygen therapy should be started at a rate of 10 L/min through a rebreathing mask, and intravenous fluids should be administered immediately for hypotension, preferably via a central venous line. Medical therapy should begin with epinephrine, which is the drug of choice for severe allergic reactions to contrast media. Epinephrine increases blood pressure by causing arteriolar and venous vasoconstriction via α-receptor stimulation. It also activates β1 receptors, which causes increased myocardial contractility and is responsible for increased heart rate. Epinephrine activation of β2 receptors leads to bronchodilation, which relieves severe bronchospasm that can occur in acute severe reactions to contrast media. Epinephrine 1:1000 dilution subcutaneously at a dose of 0.1 to 0.3 mL should be given immediately. If there is severe bronchospasm or airway compromise a more dilute solution of epinephrine, 1:10,000, can be given at a dose of 1 to 3 mL (0.1–0.3 mg) intravenously, preferably via a central line.[20] In patients with moderate symptomatic bronchospasm without hypotension, an inhaled bronchodilator such as nebulized albuterol can also be given for severe bronchospasm. High-dose intravenous steroids should also be considered at the time of acute severe reactions. The onset of action for steroids is not immediate and can take several hours to be effective; therefore, there is little to no effect on the initial signs and symptoms of acute reactions to contrast media. However, steroids have also been shown to stabilize cell membranes and prevent the biphasic anaphylaxis reaction that can occur from several hours up to 72 hours after acute severe allergic reactions.[21]

As already discussed, to initiate appropriate therapy it is important to distinguish these reactions from vasodepressor responses. Whereas observation and intravascular volume replacement using intravenous fluids are the common and first steps in both situations, pharmacologic therapy is drastically different. In severe vasodepressor response, atropine, a competitive inhibitor of acetylcholine, is the drug of choice for reversing bradycardia. Atropine, 1 mg intravenously should be given immediately, and vital signs should be monitored closely. Repeat administration of atropine, 0.8 to 1 mg intravenously can be given every 3 to 5 minutes up to a total of 3 mg in adults.[10]

DELAYED REACTIONS

Delayed adverse events occur from 60 minutes to 7 days after exposure to contrast media. These delayed reactions are usually mild in comparison with the acute allergic-like reactions and mainly include maculopapular rash, erythema, urticaria, and, rarely, angioedema. Most patients with delayed cutaneous reactions present with macular or maculopapular exanthema. The symmetric drug-related intertriginous and flexural exanthema (SDRIFE) and drug-related eosinophilia with systemic symptoms (DRESS) are specific exanthemas common to delayed cutaneous reactions to contrast media (**Fig. 2**).[22]

The incidence of delayed adverse events to contrast media has been reported as up to 14% in some studies.[23] Most of these reactions are thought to be T-cell mediated, and skin biopsies have shown T-cell infiltrate in the dermis.[24,25] Prior immunotherapy for certain malignancies using recombinant interleukin-2 agents has also been shown to increase the frequency of delayed reactions to iodinated contrast, owing to stimulation of T lymphocytes. One prospective study found that 11.8% of patients receiving interleukin-2 therapy developed delayed reaction to intravenous contrast, compared with 3.9% in those not receiving interleukin-2.[26]

A history of allergic reactions also increases the likelihood of a delayed reaction by a factor of 2, and a previous reaction to contrast medium can increase the risk of late reaction by a factor of 1.7 to 3.3.[24] The development of delayed cutaneous

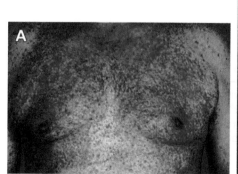
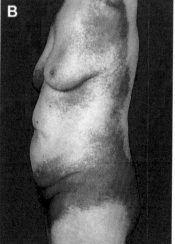

Fig. 2. Typical appearance of maculopapular exanthema (*A*) and symmetric drug-related intertriginous and flexural exanthema (*B*) associated with delayed cutaneous reactions to contrast media. (*From* Brockow K. Immediate and delayed cutaneous reactions to radiocontrast media. Chem Immunol Allergy 2012;97:184; with permission.)

reactions may also be related to the contrast agent being used. The use of iso-osmolar contrast agents is associated with a 3-times greater risk of developing a delayed cutaneous reaction than with the use of low-osmolar contrast agents.[27] Delayed reactions are usually self-limited and the treatment of delayed reactions is based on symptom management, which includes oral antihistamines, emollients, and topical steroids. Persistent delayed reactions that do not resolve with standard treatment may necessitate further consultation with a dermatologist or allergist.

It is important to consider delayed reactions to contrast when patients report maculopapular rashes several days after contrast-based procedures. It is not infrequent that the results of the procedure had prompted the initiation of other pharmacologic therapies and that the reactions are related to the pharmacologic agents rather than the contrast exposure days earlier. A commonly encountered clinical scenario is patients receiving P2Y12 inhibitors such as clopidogrel after undergoing coronary angiography and stenting. In these settings, and if the reaction is reasonably tolerated, it is prudent to consider a delayed reaction to contrast and continue using the prescribed drugs for a few days, during which the reaction would most commonly subside. If the skin manifestations do not subside within a few days, one must consider the possibility of a reaction to the prescribed drug and instruct the patient to discontinue it while prescribing an alternative.

In difficult clinical situations, skin-patch and delayed intradermal testing can also be used to confirm the diagnosis of delayed reactions related to contrast media, with delayed intradermal testing being more sensitive.[6] Because there is high cross-reactivity between different contrast media, patch testing or delayed intradermal testing should also include different contrast media to assess for negative reactions to help identify 1 or more contrast media that can be tolerated with future exposure.

PREVENTION OF CONTRAST REACTIONS
Identifying the Susceptible Patient

Prevention of adverse reactions associated with contrast media begins by recognizing those who are at an increased risk for developing adverse reactions. Although there is no guarantee that a patient is completely immune from developing such reactions, some patients should be considered high risk, and targeted for preventive measures. The most significant predictor of an adverse reaction to contrast is history of an adverse reaction during a prior exposure. Patients with such history have a 17% to 35% risk of a recurrent reaction with a second contrast exposure. Patients with atopic conditions, such as asthma and allergic rhinitis, are also at higher risk. Those with asthma have a risk that is approximately 6 times that of the general population. A history of allergic reactions to seafood or shellfish was once thought to be a risk factor for the development of anaphylactoid reactions to iodinated contrast. However, there was no associated increased risk when compared with persons with other food allergies.[28,29] Box 1 summarizes the predisposing risk factors that are commonly considered before contrast exposure.

Pharmacologic Preventive Regimens

Several regimens of premedication have been used to lower the risk of repeat adverse reactions; however, the optimal approach has not been defined. The most common method to premedication includes the use of corticosteroids and antihistamines. Corticosteroids are thought to stabilize the cell membrane through a complex signaling mechanism that results in an increased formation of C1 esterase, ultimately leading to the inhibition of bradykinin, leukotrienes, and other inflammatory mediators responsible for anaphylactoid reactions.[30] The use of antihistamines has also been shown to reduce pruritus, flushing, and cough by inhibiting the release of proinflammatory cytokines. Whereas the effects of corticosteroids on membrane stabilization can take up to 12 hours to reach peak effect, H1-antihistamine effects are more rapid, with peak effect occurring within 30 minutes to 2 hours. Based on several studies,[31,32] the most widely used pretreatment regimen includes the use of oral prednisone, 50 mg at 13 hours, 7 hours, and 1 hour before contrast

---

Box 1
Patients at higher risk for development of contrast reactions

1. History of previous anaphylactoid reactions
2. History of atopic conditions such as bronchial asthma, allergic rhinitis, and/or other allergic conditions
3. History of food or medication allergy
4. History of interleukin-2 therapy
5. Hematologic disorders (myeloma, polycythemia, sickle cell disease)
6. Concurrent medications (β-blockers, nonsteroidal anti-inflammatories)
7. Females (risk higher than males)

Table 3
Pretreatment regimens for patients with prior anaphylactoid contrast reactions

Elective or Nonurgent Procedures	Emergent Procedures
Oral prednisone, 50 mg at 13 h, 7 h, and 1 h before exposure to contrast	Option 1 Most Appropriate Methylprednisolone, 40 mg or hydrocortisone, 200 mg intravenously immediately and every 4 h until contrast exposure and Diphenhydramine, 50 mg IV 1 h before contrast administration
And Diphenhydramine, 50 mg oral, IV or IM 1 h before exposure to contrast	Option 2 History of allergy to methylprednisolone, aspirin, or NSAIDs, especially if asthmatic Dexamethasone, 7.5 mg IV or betamethasone, 6 mg IV immediately and every 4 h until contrast exposure and Diphenhydramine, 50 mg IV 1 h before contrast administration
Alternative (for patients not able to receive oral medications) IV methylprednisolone, 40 mg at 13 h, 7 h, and 1 h before exposure to contrast	Option 3 Omit steroids (inadequate time interval for corticosteroid effect) Diphenhydramine, 50 mg IV only, immediately before contrast administration

Abbreviations: IM, intramuscularly; IV, intravenously; NSAID, nonsteroidal anti-inflammatory drug.
   Data from American College of Radiology Committee on Drugs and Contrast Media. ACR manual on contrast media. 9th edition. Reston (VA): American College of Radiology; 2013. p. 6–11; with permission.

injection along with diphenhydramine, 50 mg 1 hour before contrast injection. For patients who have had intermediate to severe anaphylactoid reactions to high-osmolar ionic contrast, a nonionic low-osmolar or iso-osmolar contrast should be considered for repeat examinations.[33]

Patients with a prior intermediate or severe reaction to contrast media who require an emergent cardiac catheterization require special attention and consideration before contrast exposure. To date, no studies have shown that the short-term use of corticosteroids prevent or decrease the risk of anaphylactoid reactions to contrast media. The effects of corticosteroids may be seen within 1 hour of administration; however, the main effects of corticosteroids on circulating mast cells, basophils, and histamine were seen in 4 to 6 hours based on experimental data.[34–36] When contrast exposure cannot be delayed (eg, in a setting of acute myocardial infarction requiring emergent angioplasty) to allow time for corticosteroids to reach peak effect, some consider only using diphenhydramine, 50 mg intravenously at the time of contrast exposure for emergency procedures. However, it should be noted that the use of H1-antihistaminic agents alone have not been proved to prevent severe anaphylactoid reactions. The premedication regimens for nonemergent and emergent procedures recommended by the American College of Radiology *Manual on Contrast Media* (version 9, 2013) procedures are presented in **Table 3**.[37]

REFERENCES

1. McClennan BL. Ionic and nonionic iodinated contrast media: evaluation and strategies for use. AJR Am J Roentgenol 1990;155(2):225–33.
2. Morcos SK, Thomsen HS. Adverse reactions to iodinated contrast media. Eur Radiol 2001;11:1267–75.
3. Nissen SE, Douglas JS, Dreifus LS, et al. Use of nonionic or low osmolar contrast agents in cardiovascular procedures. J Am Coll Cardiol 1993;21:269–73.
4. Zuckerman LS, Frichliing TD, Wolf NM, et al. Effect of calcium-binding additives on ventricular fibrillation and repolarization changes during coronary angiography. J Am Coll Cardiol 1987;10:1249–53.
5. Meth MJ, Maibach HI. Current understanding of contrast media reactions and implications for clinical management. Drug Saf 2006;29(2):133–41.
6. Brockow K, Christiansen C, Kanny G, et al. Management of hypersensitivity reactions to iodinated contrast media. Allergy 2005;60:150–8.
7. Katayama H, Yamaguchi K, Kozuka T, et al. Adverse reactions to ionic and nonionic contrast media. A report from the Japanese Committee on the Safety of Contrast Media. Radiology 1990;175:621–8.
8. Wolf GL, Arenson RL, Cross AP. A prospective trial of ionic vs nonionic contrast agents in routine clinical

practice: comparison of adverse effects. Am J Roentgenol 1989;152:939–44.

9. Caro JJ, Trindade E, McGregor M. The risks of death and of severe nonfatal reactions with high- vs low-osmolality contrast media: a meta-analysis. Am J Roentgenol 1991;156:825–32.

10. Bush WH, Swanson DP. Acute reactions to intravascular contrast media: types, risk factors, recognition, and specific treatment. AJR Am J Roentgenol 1991; 157:1153–61.

11. Mita H, Tadokoro K, Akiyama K. Detection of IgE antibody to a radio- contrast medium. Allergy 1998;53:1133–40.

12. Kanny G, Maria Y, Mentre B, et al. Case report: recurrent anaphylactic shock to radiographic contrast media. Evidence supporting an exceptional IgE-mediated reaction. Allerg Immunol 1993;25:425–30.

13. Dewachter P, Mouton-Faivre C, Felden F. Allergy and contrast media. Allergy 2001;56:250–1.

14. Laroche D, Vergnaud MC, Sillard B, et al. Biochemical markers of anaphylactoid reactions to drugs. Comparison of plasma histamine and tryptase. Anesthesiology 1991;75:945–9.

15. Trcka J, Schmidt C, Seitz CS, et al. Anaphylaxis to iodinated contrast material: nonallergic hypersensitivity or IgE-mediated allergy? AJR Am J Roentgenol 2008;190:666.

16. Brockow K, Romano A, Aberer W, et al. Skin testing in patients with hypersensitivity reactions to iodinated contrast media—a European multicenter study. Allergy 2009;64:234.

17. Laroche D, Namour F, Lefrancois C, et al. Anaphylactoid and anaphylactic reactions to iodinated contrast material. Allergy 1999;54:13–6.

18. Goss JE, Chambers CE, Heupler FA. Systemic anaphylactoid reactions to iodinated contrast media during cardiac catheterization procedures: guidelines for prevention, diagnosis, and treatment. Cathet Cardiovasc Diagn 1995;34(2):99–104.

19. American College of Radiology Committee on Drugs and Contrast Media. ACR manual on contrast media. 5th edition. Reston (VA): American College of Radiology; 2004. p. 5–77.

20. Cochran ST. Anaphylactoid reactions to radiocontrast media. Curr Allergy Asthma Rep 2005;5:28–31.

21. Tole JW, Lieberman P. Biphasic anaphylaxis: review of incidence, clinical predictors, and observation recommendations. Immunol Allergy Clin North Am 2007;27(2):309–26.

22. Brockow K. Immediate and delayed cutaneous reactions to radiocontrast media. Chem Immunol Allergy 2012;97:180–90.

23. Loh S, Bagheri S, Katzberg RW, et al. Delayed adverse reaction to contrast-enhanced CT: a prospective single-center study comparison to control group without enhancement. Radiology 2010;255(3):764–71.

24. Bellin MF, Stacul F, Webb JA, et al. Late adverse reactions to intravascular iodine based contrast media: an update. Eur Radiol 2011;21:2305–10.

25. Kanny G, Pichler W, Morisset M, et al. T-cell mediated reactions to iodinated contrast media: evaluation by skin and lymphocyte activations tests. J Allergy Clin Immunol 2005;115:179–85.

26. Choyke PL, Miller DL, Lotze MT, et al. Delayed reactions to contrast media after interleukin-2 immunotherapy. Radiology 1992;183(1):111–4.

27. Sutton AG, Finn P, Grech ED, et al. Early and late reactions after the use of iopamidol 340, ioxaglate 320, and iodixanol 320 in cardiac catheterization. Am Heart J 2001;141(4):677–81.

28. Beary A, Lieberman P, Slavin R. Seafood allergy and radiocontrast media: are physicians propagating a myth? Am J Med 2008;121:158.

29. Lang DM, Alpern MB, Visintainer PF, et al. Increased risk for anaphylactoid reaction from contrast media in patients on beta-adrenergic blockers or with asthma. Ann Intern Med 1991;115(4):270–6.

30. Lasser EC, Lang JH, Lyon SG, et al. Glucocorticoid-induced elevations of C1-esterase inhibitor: a mechanism for protection against lethal dose range contrast challenge in rabbits. Invest Radiol 1981; 16:20–3.

31. Marshall GD Jr, Lieberman PL. Comparison of three pretreatment protocols to prevent anaphylactoid reactions to radiocontrast media. Ann Allergy 1991;67:70.

32. Greenberger PA, Patterson R. The prevention of immediate generalized reactions to radiocontrast media in high-risk patients. J Allergy Clin Immunol 1991;87:867.

33. Bertrand ME, Esplugas E, Piessens J, et al. Influence of a nonionic, iso-osmolar contrast medium (iodixanol) versus an ionic, low-osmolar contrast medium (ioxaglate) on major adverse cardiac events in patients undergoing percutaneous transluminal coronary angioplasty. Circulation 2000;101(2): 131–6.

34. Saavedra-Delgado AM, Mathews KP, Pan PM, et al. Dose-response studies of the suppression of whole blood histamine and basophil counts by prednisone. J Allergy Clin Immunol 1980;66(6):464–71.

35. Lasser EC. Pretreatment with corticosteroids to prevent reactions to IV contrast: overview and implications. AJR Am J Roentgenol 1988;150:257–9.

36. Miura T, Inagaki N, Yoshida K, et al. Mechanisms for glucocorticoid inhibition of immediate hypersensitivity reactions in rats. Jpn J Pharmacol 1992; 59(1):77–87.

37. American College of Radiology Committee on Drugs and Contrast Media. ACR manual on contrast media. 9th edition. Reston (VA): American College of Radiology; 2013. p. 6–11.

Relative Nephrotoxicity of Different Contrast Media

 CrossMark

Iram Aqeel, MD, Amarinder S. Garcha, MD,
Michael R. Rudnick, MD*

KEYWORDS

- Nephrotoxicity • Contrast media • Contrast-induced nephropathy • Osmolar contrast agent

KEY POINTS

- Contrast-induced nephropathy (CIN) is a common cause of acute kidney injury in hospitalized patients and is associated with increased morbidity and mortality, especially in those who require dialysis.
- Although osmolality is an important factor in causing CIN, other mechanisms contribute to the pathogenesis of CIN.
- Clinical studies show no difference between iso-osmolar and low-osmolar agents in terms of nephrotoxicity, except for iohexol and ioxaglate, which may be more nephrotoxic compared with other low-osmolar agents.

INTRODUCTION

Contrast-induced nephropathy (CIN) is a common problem, especially in the inpatient setting. Depending on patient characteristics, the incidence of CIN is reported to be as high as 31%.[1]

Contrast-induced nephropathy is traditionally defined as an absolute increase in serum creatinine by 0.5 mg/dL or a relative increase by 25% from baseline, after exposure to contrast media. The serum creatinine level usually increases within 24 to 48 hours after contrast administration, peaks at 3 to 5 days, and returns to baseline in 1 to 3 weeks. Rarely, in severe cases, temporary or sometimes permanent renal replacement therapy may be needed. CIN is associated with increased mortality, especially when CIN requires dialysis. The incidence of CIN depends on several factors, some of which are patient-related, whereas others are procedure-related. Among patient-related factors, underlying chronic kidney disease (CKD) and diabetes mellitus are the most important. Procedure-related factors include type of radiologic procedure, choice of contrast agent, and the dose administered. This article describes the different types of contrast agents and compares their nephrotoxicities.

TYPES OF CONTRAST MEDIA

Depending on their osmolality relative to plasma, contrast agents are classified as high-osmolar contrast media (HOCM), low-osmolar contrast media (LOCM), or iso-osmolar contrast media (IOCM). These agents consist of either a single benzene ring (monomer) or 2 benzene rings (dimer), and can be ionic or nonionic.

First-generation contrast agents are HOCM. They are monomers that ionize in solution. Their osmolality is approximately 1400 to 1800 mOsm/kg.

Disclosures: Michael Rudnick received monies in the past from General Electric Healthcare (last honorarium 2007) and from Bracco (last honorarium 2010) for lectures, consulting, and research grants.
Renal, Electrolyte and Hypertension Division, University of Pennsylvania, 3400 Spruce Street, One Founders, Philadelphia, PA 19104, USA
* Corresponding author. Renal, Electrolyte and Hypertension Division, Penn Presbyterian Medical Center, Medical Office Building Suite 240, 39th and Market Street, Philadelphia, PA 19104.
E-mail address: Michael.rudnick@uphs.upenn.edu

Diatrizoate is an example of HOCM. These agents are rarely used for studies requiring intravascular administration, having been replaced with LOCM and IOCM, largely because of lower nephrotoxicity.

Second-generation agents are LOCM. They are also monomers. Their osmolality is 500 to 850 mOsm/kg. Contrary to what their name suggests, these agents still have a higher osmolality relative to plasma. Members of this class include agents that are nonionic and ionic (eg, ioxaglate).

The most recent class of agents are IOCMs, which are nonionic dimers with osmolality approximately equal to that of plasma (290 mOsm/kg), and hence are iso-osmolar and have the lowest osmolality compared with the previous generations. Currently, iodixanol is the only iso-osmolar contrast agent available commercially in the United States.

Fig. 1 describes the chemical structure of different contrast media. **Table 1** summarizes the different contrast agents, their brand names, and their osmolality.

ROLE OF OSMOLALITY IN THE PATHOGENESIS OF CIN

Different hypotheses exist regarding the pathogenesis of CIN. Most of the evidence comes from animal models. The most accepted explanation is that contrast media cause vasoconstriction via release of vasoconstrictors, such as endothelin and adenosine, which in the presence of already compromised renal hemodynamics cause medullary ischemia.[2] Injury to tubular epithelium seems to be mediated by reactive oxygen species.[3]

Based on clinical observations that LOCM are less nephrotoxic than HOCM, and mixed observations about the relative nephrotoxicity of LOCM to IOCM (see later discussion), the role of the osmolality of the contrast media in the pathogenesis of CIN has been debated extensively. Experimental studies have examined the effect of osmolality on degree of apoptosis in a renal epithelial cell line using DNA fragmentation as a marker. In these studies, salt and mannitol solutions with osmolality comparable to that of HOCM did not cause as much DNA fragmentation as HOCM, suggesting a direct toxic effect on the renal epithelial cells that is unique to contrast media. Subsequent studies have also elegantly demonstrated mitochondrial dysfunction at the cellular level with contrast agents but not with equiosmolar mannitol, further supporting additional mechanisms of renal injury independent of osmolality. In some animal models, IOCM have actually been shown to be more nephrotoxic than HOCM and LOCM, a finding that has been attributed to increased viscosity and tubular hydrostatic pressures.[2] The relationship of increased viscosity and nephrotoxicity has also been shown in studies using laser Doppler flow measurements, showing a greater reduction in medullary blood flow when exposed to IOCM compared with HOCM and LOCM.

Dickenmann and colleagues[4] described the phenomenon of osmotic nephrosis, a morphologic

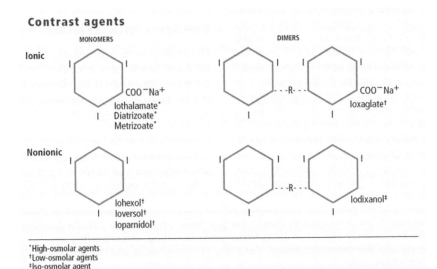

Fig. 1. Chemical structure of different contrast media. I, iodine; R, side chain. (*From* Rudnick MR, Kesselheim A, Goldfarb S. Contrast-induced nephropathy: how it develops, how to prevent it. Cleve Clin J Med 2006;73(1): 75–80, 83–7; and *Adapted from* Rudnick MR. The role of osmolality in contrast-associated nephrotoxicity. Applications in imaging—cardiac interventions. Scotch Plains (NY): Anderson Publishing; 2003.)

Table 1
Brand names and osmolality of different contrast agents

Generic Name	Brand Name	Manufacturer Name	Compound	Type	Osmolality (mOsm/kg)
Diatrizoate	Hypaque 50	Bracco Diagnostic Inc	Ionic	Monomer	1500
Metrizoate	Isopaque 370	Hangzhou Zhenghan	Ionic	Monomer	2100
Ioxaglate	Hexabrix	Guerbet LLC	Ionic	Dimer	580
Iopamidol	Isovue 370	Brighstone Pharma	Nonionic	Monomer	796
Iohexol	Omnipaque 350	GE healthcare	Nonionic	Monomer	884
Iopromide	Ultravist 370	Bayer Healthcare Pharmaceuticals	Nonionic	Monomer	774
Ioversol	Optiray 300	Mallinckrodt Inc	Nonionic	Monomer	702
Iodixanol	Visipaque	GE healthcare	Nonionic	Dimer	290

pattern of injury that involves swelling and vacuolization of proximal renal tubular cells associated with contrast media. HOCM and LOCM have been shown to cause osmotic nephrosis in rats.[4] IOCM, when used in large doses, also had the potential to cause osmotic nephrosis. Whether this histologic phenomenon contributes to permanent renal impairment is unclear.

HOCM VERSUS LOCM

High osmolar agents have been used for many decades, and their side effects, including nephrotoxicity, are well described. In the mid-1980s, with introduction of LOCM, several studies were published comparing the nephrotoxicities of LOCM and HOCM.

In 1989, Schwab and colleagues[5] conducted a prospective, randomized, double-blind, controlled trial consisting of 443 patients undergoing cardiac catheterization. The patients were divided into low-risk and high-risk groups depending on the presence of diabetes mellitus, heart failure, and CKD. The incidence of CIN was 10.2% in the diatrizoate (an HCOM) group compared with 8.2% in the iopamidol (an LOCM) group. This difference was not statistically significant. Even in the high-risk group, the incidence of CIN was 17% and 15% with diatrizoate and iopamidol, respectively, which was not statistically significant. A major limitation of this study was the small number of patients with preexisting CKD.

The first evidence that LOCM are less nephrotoxic than HOCM came from Rudnick and colleagues[6] in 1995 from a double-blind prospective trial in which 1196 patients were randomized into 4 different groups: patients with CKD with or without diabetes and those with normal kidney function with or without diabetes. Iohexol (an

LOCM) was compared with diatrizoate (an HCOM). In this study, iohexol was associated with less nephrotoxicity in patients with underlying CKD, both with and without diabetes. No difference in nephrotoxicity was seen between iohexol and diatrizoate in patients with normal kidney function, with or without diabetes. Among patients with CKD without diabetes, the incidence of CIN in patients treated with diatrizoate was 7% compared with 4% in the iohexol group. Among patients with CKD and diabetes, the incidence increased to 27% in the diatrizoate group and 12% in the iohexol group.

A meta-analysis consisting of 25 randomized controlled trials by Barrett and Carlisle[7] in 1993 supported the findings by Rudnick and colleagues.[6] In this meta-analysis, the odds of CIN was 0.61 times greater with LOCM than with HOCM. This effect was more pronounced in patients with underlying CKD.

Over the course of time, the cost difference between LOCM and HOCM disappeared and the use of LOCM, because of the lower nephrotoxicity and reduced systemic side effects, became the standard of care.

LOCM VERSUS IOCM

With the introduction of IOCM in the mid-1990s, it was speculated that with an osmolality close to that of plasma, these agents would be less nephrotoxic than LOCM in high-risk patients, similar to the reduction in CIN seen with the introduction of LOCM. Many studies have compared LOCM and IOCM in different radiographic procedures. These studies can be divided into intra-arterial studies, such as coronary or aortofemoral angiography, and intravenous studies, such as primarily computed tomography (CT).

INTRA-ARTERIAL STUDIES: COMPARING THE IOCM IODIXANOL WITH DIFFERENT LOCM

In 2003, Aspelin and colleagues[8] published the NEPHRIC trial. This trial was a randomized, double-blind, prospective multicenter study of 129 patients with diabetes and a mean creatinine level between 1.5 to 3.5 mg/dL undergoing coronary or aortofemoral angiography. The study compared iodixanol (an IOCM) with iohexol (an LOCM) and showed that the incidences of CIN were 3% and 26%, respectively ($P = .002$). The odds ratio for CIN in the iodixanol group compared with the iohexol group was 0.09.

These results were confirmed by the RECOVER trial reported by Jo and colleagues[9] in 2006, which compared iodixanol with ioxaglate (an LOCM), an ionic dimeric compound, in 300 patients undergoing coronary angiography with or without percutaneous coronary intervention. The incidence of CIN was 17.0% in the ioxaglate group compared with 7.9% in the iodixanol group ($P = .021$). The odds ratio for CIN for iodixanol compared with ioxaglate was 0.41. The investigators also showed that the incidence of CIN in subgroups of patients with severe CKD (creatinine clearance <30 mL/min) was significantly lower in the iodixanol group (12.5% vs 53.3%). Similarly, among patients with diabetes, the incidence of CIN was 10.4% in the iodixanol group and 26.5% in the ioxaglate group.

The CARE trial reported by Solomon and colleagues[10] in 2007 showed contrary findings. This multicenter, randomized, double-blind controlled trial consisted of 414 patients with moderate to severe CKD (glomerular filtration rate [GFR], 20–59 mL/min) undergoing cardiac angiography. This study compared iodixanol and iopamidol. The incidence of CIN was 6.7% and 4.4%, respectively ($P = .39$). In the subgroup of patients with diabetes and CKD, the incidence of CIN was 5.1% in the iopamidol group compared with 13% in the iodixanol group ($P = .11$). The investigators concluded that no significant difference was seen between iodixanol and iopamidol in the occurrence of CIN in patients with CKD with or without diabetes.

In 2008, Rudnick and colleagues[11] published the VALOR trial comparing iodixanol with another LOCM (ie, ioversol). It was a prospective, double-blind trial of 299 patients undergoing coronary angiography with mean baseline creatinine level of 1.9 mg/dL. The incidence of CIN in the iodixanol group was 21.8%, which was not statistically different from 23.8% in the ioversol group ($P = .78$). In 2009, Laskey and colleagues[12] conducted a prospective, randomized, controlled trial comparing iodixanol and iopamidol in patients with CKD

undergoing coronary angiography. The incidence of CIN was 11.2% in the iodixanol group compared with 9.8% in the iopamidol group ($P = .7$). These studies suggest that there is no difference in the incidence of CIN between iodixanol and some of the specific LOCM.

INTRAVENOUS STUDIES: COMPARING THE IOCM IODIXANOL WITH DIFFERENT LOCM

Until 2008, most published studies evaluating the incidence of CIN focused on intra-arterial administration of contrast agents in patients with renal insufficiency.[8–11] Several studies have now compared the incidence of CIN after intravenous use of iodixanol and various LOCM.[13–16]

In the 2006 randomized, double-blind, controlled IMAPCT trial comparing CT with either iodixanol or iopamidol (LOCM) in 153 patients with CKD (GFR <60 mL/min), Barrett and colleagues[13] reported an incidence of CIN (defined as an absolute increase of 0.5 mg/dL in creatinine) of 2.6% in the iodixanol group and 0% in the iopamidol group ($P = .2$).

The PREDICT trial[14] reported by Kuhn and colleagues in 2008 studied the patient population at highest risk for CIN (ie, patients with CKD and diabetes). This randomized double-blind trial compared iodixanol with iopamidol in 248 patients undergoing CT who had moderate to severe CKD (glomerular filtration rate 29–59 mL/min) and diabetes. The incidence of CIN was 5.6% in the iopamidol group and 4.9% in the iodixanol group, which was not statistically significant. No difference in the incidence of CIN was seen in subset high-risk groups (ie, patients with advanced CKD with GFR <40 mL/min and those receiving >140 mL of contrast agent).

Concurrently, Thomsen and colleagues[15] reported on the ACTIVE trial, a multicenter, randomized, double-blind study comparing iodixanol with iomeprol (LOCM) in148 patients with CKD undergoing CT, which showed that the incidence of CIN was actually higher in the iodixanol group (6.9% vs 0%; $P<.05$).

Also in 2008, Nguyen and colleagues[16] conducted a single-center, randomized, double-blind study comparing iodixanol and iopromide in 117 patients with CKD undergoing CT. The incidence of CIN in the iodixanol group was 8.5% compared with 27.8% the iopromide group ($P = .012$), a finding that is inconsistent with the studies described previously.

In 2009, Bruce and colleagues[17] conducted a retrospective study on more than 11,000 patients divided into 3 groups: those receiving intravenous iohexol, those receiving intravenous iodixanol, and a control group that underwent unenhanced CT. The incidence of acute kidney injury (AKI) was similar among all 3 groups for baseline creatinine values up to 1.8 mg/dL. With creatinine more than 1.8 mg/dL, the incidence of AKI was highest in iohexol group.

Table 2 summarizes the larger studies that compared CIN incidence between LOCM and IOCM vis intra-arterial and intravenous administration.

COMPARISON OF CIN INCIDENCE BETWEEN DIFFERENT LOCM AND IOCM

The NEPHRIC and RECOVER trials show that iodixanol is less nephrotoxic than LOCM, whereas the IMPACT, CARE, VALOR, PREDICT, and ACTIVE trials showed no difference in nephrotoxicity. Although some of the inconsistencies among these studies can be explained by differences in study design and population, some investigators postulate that the specific LOCM iohexol, used in the NEPHRIC study, may be more nephrotoxic than other LOCM. This conclusion was reported in 2009 by Heinrich and colleagues[18] in their meta-analysis of 25 prospective, randomized, controlled trials comparing iodixanol and various LOCM in a total of more than 3000 patients. Of these trials, 17 included patients with intra-arterial contrast administration, with intravenous administration used in the remainder. When all studies were pooled together, no difference in the risk of CIN was seen between iodixanol and other LOCM (relative risk [RR], 0.80; $P = .1$). In the intravenous subgroup, reduction in CIN risk was not found with iodixanol compared with other LOCM (RR, 1.08; $P = .79$), not even in high-risk patients with underlying CKD and diabetes. However, among intra-arterial studies, iodixanol was associated with reduced risk of CIN in patients with underlying CKD when compared with iohexol (RR, 0.38; $P<.01$). However, this protective effect of iodixanol disappeared when compared with other noniohexol LOCM.

A similar meta-analysis reported by From and colleagues[19] in 2010 included 36 randomized controlled trials comparing iodixanol and LOCM. A statistically significant reduction in CIN risk was found in the iodixanol group only when compared with iohexol (odds ratio, 0.25; $P<.001$) and not with other LOCM.

Although any differences in nephrotoxicity between iohexol and the other LOCM can only be proven by a study directly comparing iohexol and another specific LOCM (to date none has been performed), these findings support the possibility that all LOCM may not have similar renal safety.

Some investigators have postulated that viscosity along with osmolality may play a role in nephrotoxicity. Several experimental studies suggest that the increased viscosity of iodixanol, resulting from its dimeric composition, contributes to this contrast agent's nephrotoxicity. High viscosity leads to increased red blood cell aggregation, causing stasis in renal tubules, leading to tubular ischemia. Lancelot and colleagues[20] showed that iodixanol caused significantly more medullary hypoperfusion than ioxaglate in the dog kidney. Similarly, Seeliger and colleagues[21] compared the high-osmolar substances iopromide and mannitol to the high-viscous substances iodixanol and dextran in rats. The high-viscosity group demonstrated more medullary hypoperfusion and increases in serum creatinine than the animals treated with high-osmolar compounds. These experimental studies suggest that, despite a lower osmolality, the risk of CIN with IOCM may be higher than with LOCM. The clinical significance of these findings is unclear, because clinical studies have shown either a reduced or equal CIN incidence with IOCM and LOCM.

Some studies have compared the incidence of CIN associated with LOCM and IOCM in low-risk patients (ie, those with an estimated GFR of approximately $\geq$60 mL/min). These studies can be appropriately criticized that the inability to show a CIN difference between LOCM and IOCM is because of the extremely low incidence of CIN, regardless of contrast choice, in low-risk patients. However, the studies in **Table 2** and the cited meta-analyses[18,19] are primarily in high-risk patients, and as stated did not show any difference in CIN risk between IOCM and LOCM except when the LOCM was iohexol or ioxaglate. These observations thus negate the criticism of studies that have compared CIN from IOCM and LOCM in mostly low-risk patients. In contrast, very few data compare IOCM and LOCM in very high-risk individual patients, such as those with stage 4 (estimated GFR <30 mL/min) or worse CKD. Whether IOCM would have a higher, equal, or lower incidence of CIN in these very high-risk patients remains unknown. Fortunately, these patients constitute only a small percentage of patients who require cardiac angiography. The authors' practice is to use selected LOCM for all patients, regardless of how low the GFR is, recognizing that the choice to use IOCM solely in these very high-risk patients would not be inappropriate based on current data.

CURRENT PRACTICE AND GUIDELINES

The 2012 Kidney Disease: Improving Global Outcomes (KDIGO) Clinical Practice Guideline for

Table 2
Randomized control trials comparing iodixanol and low-osmolar contrast agents

Author, Year	Type of Study	Type of LOCM	Type of Procedure	N	Incidence of CIN (Iodixanol) (%)	Incidence of CIN (LOCM) (%)	P Value
Aspelin et al,[8] 2003	Multicenter, randomized, double-blind NEPHRIC trial	Iodixanol vs iohexol	Coronary or aortofemoral angiography	129	3.0	26.0	.002
Jo et al,[9] 2006	Single-center, randomized, double-blind RECOVER trial	Iodixanol vs ioxaglate	Coronary angiography with or without percutaneous intervention	300	7.9	17.0	.021
Barrett et al,[13] 2006	Multicenter, randomized, double-blind, IMPACT trial	Iodixanol vs iopamidol	CT	153	2.6	0	.200
Solomon et al,[10] 2007	Multicenter, randomized, double-blind CARE trial	Iodixanol vs iopamidol	Coronary angiography	414	6.7	4.4	.390
Rudnick et al,[11] 2008	Multi- centered, randomized, double blind VALOR trial	Iodixanol vs ioversal	Coronary angiography	299	21.8	23.8	.780
Kuhn et al,[14] 2008	Multicenter, randomized, double-blind PREDICT trial	Iodixanol vs iopamidol	CT	248	4.9	5.6	1.000
Nguyen et al,[16] 2008	Single-center, randomized, double-blind	Iodixanol vs iopromide	CT	117	8.5	27.8	.012
Thomsen et al,[15] 2008	Multicenter, randomized, double-blind ACTIVE trial	Iodixanol vs iomeprol	CT	148	6.9	0	<.050
Laskey et al,[12] 2009	Multicenter, randomized, double-blind	Iodixanol vs iopamidol	Coronary angiography	418	11.2	9.8	.700

Acute Kidney Injury recommends that CIN be defined and staged according to the KDIGO recommendation for the definition of AKI. Individuals who develop changes in kidney function after administration of intravascular contrast media should be evaluated for CIN and other possible causes of AKI.[22]

Patients who are considered for a procedure that requires intravascular administration of an iodinated contrast medium should be assessed for the risk for CIN and, in particular, screened for preexisting CKD. In patients at increased risk for CIN, alternative imaging methods should be considered. If no alternative imaging is feasible, the lowest possible dose of contrast medium should be used. Furthermore, IOCM or LOCM rather than HOCM should be used.[22] KDIGO does not specifically comment on the preferential avoidance of iohexol in a patient who is at high-risk of CIN. KDIGO also recommends intravenous volume expansion with isotonic sodium chloride or sodium bicarbonate solutions and the use of oral N-acetylcysteine (NAC) in patients at increased risk of CIN.[22]

The 2012 ACCF/AHA (American College of Cardiology Foundation/American Heart Association) updated guidelines for the management of patients with unstable angina or non–ST-elevation myocardial infarction do not recommend the use or avoidance of any particular IOCM or LOCM in view of the inconsistent relationships between the various contrast agents and CIN.[23] These guidelines, however, recommend adequate hydration before angiography, although they are silent on the choice of fluid to be used for this purpose.[23] These guidelines also note a benefit of NAC as an adjunct to hydration for preventing CIN but do not make a standing recommendation on the use of NAC.

Based on current data, the authors recommend the use of either IOCM or LOCM in patients at high-risk for CIN, but would not use either iohexol or ioxaglate if LOCM were to be used.

REFERENCES

1. Rihal CS, Textor SC, Grill DE, et al. Incidence and prognostic importance of acute renal failure after percutaneous coronary intervention. Circulation 2002;105(19):2259–64.
2. Rudnick MR, Goldfarb S. Pathogenesis of contrast-induced nephropathy: experimental and clinical observations with an emphasis on the role of osmolality. Rev Cardiovasc Med 2003;4(Suppl 5):S28–33.
3. Pisani A, Riccio E, Andreucci M, et al. Role of reactive oxygen species in pathogenesis of radiocontrast-induced nephropathy. Biomed Res Int 2013;2013:868321.
4. Dickenmann M, Oettl T, Mihatsch MJ, et al. Osmotic nephrosis: acute kidney injury with accumulation of proximal tubular lysosomes due to administration of exogenous solutes. Am J Kidney Dis 2008;51(3): 491–503.
5. Schwab SJ, Hlatky MA, Pieper KS, et al. Contrast nephrotoxicity: a randomized controlled trial of a nonionic and an ionic radiographic contrast agent. N Engl J Med 1989;320(3):149–53.
6. Rudnick MR, Goldfarb S, Wexler L, et al. Nephrotoxicity of ionic and nonionic contrast media in 1196 patients: a randomized trial. The Iohexol Cooperative Study. Kidney Int 1995;47(1):254–61.
7. Barrett BJ, Carlisle EJ. Metaanalysis of the relative nephrotoxicity of high- and low-osmolality iodinated contrast media. Radiology 1993;188(1):171–8.
8. Aspelin P, Aubry P, Fransson SG, et al. Nephrotoxic effects in high-risk patients undergoing angiography. N Engl J Med 2003;348(6):491–9.
9. Jo SH, Youn TJ, Koo BK, et al. Renal toxicity evaluation and comparison between Visipaque (iodixanol) and Hexabrix (ioxaglate) in patients with renal insufficiency undergoing coronary angiography: the RECOVER study: a randomized controlled trial. J Am Coll Cardiol 2006;48(5):924–30.
10. Solomon RJ, Natarajan MK, Doucet S, et al. Cardiac Angiography in Renally Impaired Patients (CARE) study: a randomized double-blind trial of contrast-induced nephropathy in patients with chronic kidney disease. Circulation 2007;115(25):3189–96.
11. Rudnick MR, Davidson CM, Leskey WK, et al. Nephrotoxicity of iodixanol versus ioversol in patients with chronic kidney disease: the Visipaque Angiography/Interventions with Laboratory Outcomes in Renal Insufficiency (VALOR) trial. Am Heart J 2008;156(4):776–82.
12. Laskey WK, Aspelin P, Davidson CM, et al. Nephrotoxicity of iodixanol versus iopamidol in patients with chronic kidney disease and diabetes mellitus undergoing coronary angiographic procedures. Am Heart J 2009;158(5):822–8.
13. Barrett BJ, Katzberg RW, Thomsen HS, et al. Contrast-induced nephropathy in patients with chronic kidney disease undergoing computed tomography: a double-blind comparison of iodixanol and iopamidol. Invest Radiol 2006;41(11):815–21.
14. Kuhn MJ, Chen N, Sahani DV, et al. The PREDICT study: a randomized double-blind comparison of contrast-induced nephropathy after low- or isoosmolar contrast agent exposure. AJR Am J Roentgenol 2008;191(1):151–7.
15. Thomsen HS, Morcos SK, Erley C, et al. The ACTIVE Trial: comparison of the effects on renal function of iomeprol-400 and iodixanol-320 in patients with chronic kidney disease undergoing abdominal computed tomography. Invest Radiol 2008;43(3): 170–8.

16. Nguyen SA, Suranyi P, Ravenel JG, et al. Iso-osmolality versus low-osmolality iodinated contrast medium at intravenous contrast-enhanced CT: effect on kidney function. Radiology 2008;248(1):97–105.

17. Bruce RJ, Djamali A, Shinki K, et al. Background fluctuation of kidney function versus contrast-induced nephrotoxicity. AJR Am J Roentgenol 2009;192(3):711–8.

18. Heinrich MC, Häberle L, Müller V, et al. Nephrotoxicity of iso-osmolar iodixanol compared with nonionic low-osmolar contrast media: meta-analysis of randomized controlled trials. Radiology 2009;250(1): 68–86.

19. From AM, Al Badarin FJ, McDonald FS, et al. Iodixanol versus low-osmolar contrast media for prevention of contrast induced nephropathy: meta-analysis of randomized, controlled trials. Circ Cardiovasc Interv 2010;3(4):351–8.

20. Lancelot E, Idée JM, Laclédère C, et al. Effects of two dimeric iodinated contrast media on renal medullary blood perfusion and oxygenation in dogs. Invest Radiol 2002;37(7):368–75.

21. Seeliger E, Flemming B, Wronski T, et al. Viscosity of contrast media perturbs renal hemodynamics. J Am Soc Nephrol 2007;18(11):2912–20.

22. Kellum JA, Lameire N. KDIGO clinical practice guideline for acute kidney injury. Kidney Int Suppl 2012;2(Suppl 1):8.

23. Anderson JL, Adams CD, Antman EM, et al. 2012 ACCF/AHA Focused Update Incorporated Into the ACCF/AHA 2007 Guidelines for the Management of Patients with Unstable Angina/Non-ST-Elevation Myocardial Infarction: a report of the American College of Cardiology Foundation/American Heart Association Task Force on Practice Guidelines. J Am Coll Cardiol 2013;62(11):1040–1.

Contrast-Induced Nephropathy
Definitions, Epidemiology, and Implications

Peter A. McCullough, MD, MPH, FACC, FACP, FAHA, FCCP, FNKF[a,b,*]

KEYWORDS

- Contrast-induced acute kidney injury • Serum creatinine • Chronic kidney disease • Biomarkers

KEY POINTS

- Contrast-induced acute kidney injury (CI-AKI) is defined by the Kidney Disease Global Outcomes (KDIGO) guidelines as an increase in serum creatinine of 0.3 mg/dL or greater within 48 hours of contrast use or a 50% or greater increase from baseline serum creatinine within 7 days.
- CI-AKI has been consistently associated with risk for the development of end-stage renal disease, rehospitalization for cardiac renal and other causes, and all-cause mortality.
- Reduced glomerular filtration at baseline (eGFR <60 mL/min) is the single most important risk predictor for CI-AKI, and should be a trigger for preventive measures.
- Avoidance of dehydration by using preprocedure intravenous volume expansion, particularly when the left ventricular end-diastolic pressure is low, and holding nephrotoxic drugs (nonsteroidal anti-inflammatory agents, aminoglycosides, vancomycin, calcineurin inhibitors) are the most important interventions to prevent CI-AKI.

INTRODUCTION

Contrast-induced nephropathy is now termed contrast-induced acute kidney injury (CI-AKI) to align with the Kidney Disease International Global Outcomes Guidelines (KDIGO) published in 2012.[1] Before these guidelines were created there were various terms and definitions for acute renal injury or failure, without agreement on a uniform standard. Hence the literature on the epidemiology, outcomes, and even randomized clinical trials has a plethora of inconsistent and arbitrary definitions of CI-AKI.[2] Some common definitions have included an increase level of serum creatinine (Cr) greater than 25%, 25% to 50%, greater than 50%, 50% to 100%, greater than 100%, and/or 0.5 mg/dL or higher.[3] This review summarizes the KDIGO definition as the only guidelines-proposed definition that has gone through a full consensus,

open comment period, and endorsement process. Moreover, this set of guidelines puts CI-AKI in context of other causes of AKI, including sepsis and cardiac surgery.[1]

The KDIGO definition of AKI is given in **Box 1**; **Table 1** shows the criteria for staging AKI. An increase in serum Cr of at least 0.3 mg/dL is the minimal detectable change considered above the baseline variation or noise level of this assay.[1] It is now a desired standard that all clinical laboratories use isotope dilution mass spectrophotometry (IDMS) or IDMS-traceable methods, as this is the only way of confirming Cr results between different laboratories. If there is a known time of injury, one would expect an increase of 0.3 mg/dL or more in Cr within 48 hours of the insult.[4] However, many times it is not clear when the injury occurred, and therefore, if a 1.5-fold or greater increase in Cr is seen within 7 days, this

The author has nothing to disclose.
[a] Baylor University Medical Center, Baylor Heart and Vascular Institute, Baylor Jack and Jane Hamilton Heart and Vascular Hospital, 621 North Hall Street, #H030, Dallas, TX 75226, USA; [b] The Heart Hospital, 1100 Allied Drive, Plano, TX 75093, USA
* Baylor Heart and Vascular Institute, 621 North Hall Street, #H030, Dallas, TX.
E-mail address: peteramccullough@gmail.com

interventional.theclinics.com

Box 1
Definition of acute kidney injury (AKI)

AKI is defined as any of the following

- Increase in serum creatinine by at least 0.3 mg/dL ($\geq$26.5 μmol/L) within 48 hours; or
- Increase in serum creatinine to at least 1.5 times baseline, which is known or presumed to have occurred within the prior 7 days
- Urine volume less than 0.5 mL/kg/h for 6 hours

AKI is staged according to the criteria in **Table 1**.

From Kidney Disease: Improving Global Outcomes (KDIGO) Acute Kidney Injury Work Group. KDIGO clinical practice guideline for acute kidney injury. Kidney Int 2012;Suppl 2:1–138; with permission.

---

will also meet a definition of AKI. In addition to the Cr criteria, KDIGO has also endorsed a sustained reduction in urine output of less than 0.5 mL/kg/h for at least 6 hours as another criterion to meet a definition of AKI.[1] So, for example, if a 100-kg patient had accurately measured urine output of less than 50 mL/h for 6 hours after contrast, this could meet a definition of CI-AKI. As of this writing, there are several clinical trials under way to ascertain CI-AKI using changes in both serum Cr and measured urine output, and the KDIGO definition. Thus the descriptive epidemiology described in this article relies on the older literature, which has been purely based on changes in serum Cr after exposure to iodinated contrast.

EPIDEMIOLOGY AND RISK PREDICTION

The distribution of CI-AKI and its determinants is well known. A normal human kidney has between 800,000 and 1.3 million functional nephron units. One of the most important determinants of the number of nephrons is birth weight. Lower birth weight infants start life with fewer nephrons, and

thus are at greater risk of chronic kidney disease (CKD) from a variety of diseases over time.[5] With 1.6 to 2.6 million functional nephrons in a young individual, there would need to be approximately 50% loss of function before there would be a detectable change in serum Cr. Thus, in young individuals with normal renal function there is very little chance that a significant change in serum Cr would be seen after contrast exposure. Even if contrast caused some permanent loss of renal filtration function, without a reduced mass of nephrons, CI-AKI based on a change in serum Cr would not be detectable. For this reason there are novel markers now commercially available to detect AKI without any increase in serum Cr (see later discussion).

The epidemiology and risk factors for CI-AKI thus far have been based on changes in serum Cr after contrast exposure. As a general heuristic, there needs to be an estimated glomerular filtration rate (eGFR) less than half of normal (ie, <60 mL/min/m^2, normal being 130 mL/min/m^2) before CI-AKI is observed in populations. Thus when eGFR is less than 60 mL/min/m^2 there is probably half the normal numbers of functioning nephrons, so when injury occurs there is an insufficient renal reserve to maintain filtration of creatinine at the normal rate, and one would see an increase in serum Cr of greater than 0.3 mg/dL within 48 hours. However, with the same degree of injury, if the remaining nephrons can adapt and increase their contribution to filtration, no significant change in serum Cr will be observed. Residual renal filtration function and the reserve capacity of the kidneys to respond to injury therefore account for what has been seen in the epidemiology of CI-AKI. As eGFR becomes lower in populations, there is greater certainty that Cr will increase after contrast exposure, and rates of CI-AKI will progressively increase as eGFR declines. In addition to a reduced eGFR, albuminuria, proteinuria, diabetes, heart failure, age older than 75 years, female gender, anemia, and

---

Table 1
Staging of acute kidney injury

Stage	Serum Creatinine	Urine Output
1	1.5–1.9 times baseline, or $\geq$0.3 mg/dL ($\geq$26.5 μmol/L) increase	<0.5 mL/kg/h for 6–12 h
2	2.0–2.9 times baseline	<0.5 mL/kg/h for $\geq$12 h
3	3.0 times baseline, or increase in serum creatinine to $\geq$4.0 mg/dL ($\geq$353.6 μmol/L), or initiation of renal replacement therapy, or, in patients <18 y, decrease in estimated glomerular filtration rate to <35 mL/min/1.73 m^2	<0.3 mL/kg/h for $\geq$24 h, or anuria for $\geq$12 h

From Kidney Disease: Improving Global Outcomes (KDIGO) Acute Kidney Injury Work Group. KDIGO clinical practice guideline for acute kidney injury. Kidney Int 2012;Suppl 2:1–138; with permission.

hyperglycemia have all been identified as baseline risk factors for CI-AKI.[2,6] Most of these risk factors are simply covariates for more severe baseline CKD or are mathematical elements of the eGFR equation (age, gender, race, serum Cr) preferably calculated using the CKD-EPI equation.[7] There are procedural factors that can contribute to risk including the use of high-osmolar contrast, greater contrast volumes, direct injection into the renal arteries or suprarenal aortography, cardiogenic shock, use of intra-aortic balloon counterpulsation (IABP), and transcatheter aortic valve replacement (TAVR). The contrast-related variables are related to the physiochemical properties and the quantity of iodinated contrast. In general, the higher the osmolality (particle concentration in solution), the greater is the degree of renal vasoconstriction and cellular toxicity of the agent. Osmolality cannot explain all of the toxicity because even iso-osmolar contrast causes CI-AKI, albeit at lower levels than that of high or lower osmolar contrast agents.[8] Thus, all forms of iodinated contrast have renal toxicity. The volume of contrast has been studied in many articles, and in general there is no safe "limit" for contrast volume, because at lower levels of residual eGFR smaller volumes of contrast can result in significant damage. A reasonable limit to follow can be adapted from Laskey and colleagues[9] and the National Heart Lung and Blood Institute Dynamic Registry investigators; that is, to keep the total contrast volume lower than twice the residual renal filtration value (creatinine clearance or eGFR). For example, a patient with an eGFR of 45 mL/min/1.73 m^2 should not exceed 90 mL of contrast per case in the catheterization laboratory.[9] The other procedural factors mentioned carry renal risks largely because of reductions in renal blood flow (cardiogenic shock or IABP) or because they promote superimposed atheroembolism (IABP and TAVR). It should also be mentioned that acute coronary syndromes (ACS) of all types undergoing percutaneous coronary intervention (PCI) are associated with higher rates of CI-AKI than elective coronary interventions. The reasons for this are that there may be less time for volume prophylaxis, higher degrees of neurohormonal activation, and, possibly, biochemical mediators of renal injury released in the setting of cardiac ischemia and infarction, such as catalytic or unbound iron.[10,11]

ASSOCIATION WITH ADVERSE EVENTS

There has been a consistent relationship in the literature between CI-AKI and clinically meaningful adverse and serious adverse events (SAE). It is not clear whether CI-AKI is causative or contributory, or if it is simply a marker for more severely ill patients who would incur these events after PCI irrespective of renal injury. Nevertheless, CI-AKI has been implicated as an associated factor for recurrent myocardial infarction (MI), stroke, the development of heart failure, the need for renal replacement therapy including dialysis, bleeding, longer stays in hospital, readmissions for cardiac, renal, and other causes, permanent loss of eGFR (typically considered significant if >25% loss) at 90 days, and mortality, both inpatient and longer term (**Fig. 1**).[12–14] Although death is the most important complication associated with CI-AKI and often occurs despite use of renal replacement therapy, it may be that CI-AKI is simply a marker for older more chronically ill and frail individuals who will succumb to multiorgan failure in the setting of critical illness following PCI. The Cardiac Angiography in Renally Impaired Patients (CARE) study reported on clinical outcomes of 294 of 414 (71%) subjects after 12 months of follow-up after having been randomized to iso-osmolar iodixanol or low-osmolar iopamidol during coronary angiography.[15] Of those who met a KDIGO definition of CI-AKI, the incident-rate ratio for a major cardiorenal end point include death, stroke, MI, and end-stage renal disease requiring dialysis was 3.2 (95% CI 1.1–8.7; $P = .02$ adjusted for contrast agent, age, gender, diabetes, hypertension, congestive heart failure, coronary artery disease severity, and left ventricular ejection fraction). Because of bias with respect to a large-fraction loss to follow-up, treatment inferences with respect to use of contrast agents could not be made. However, this study is yet another source of information suggesting that CI-AKI does have an independent associative relationship with major adverse renal and cardiac events. If there is a causative role of CI-AKI in cardiovascular events, it is probably in the development of heart failure. As AKI unfolds, there is neurohormonal activation, retention of salt and water, increased pressure overload, and volume overload, in addition to a CKD-related cardiomyopathy. This clinical scenario, in which heart failure is caused by AKI and whereby the AKI clearly occurred first, is now termed a type 3 cardiorenal syndrome.[16]

NOVEL BIOMARKERS AND SUBCLINICAL ACUTE KIDNEY INJURY

In recent years there has been considerable advancement in the use of biomarkers besides Cr for the detection of AKI, as shown in **Fig. 2**. At the time of writing, there is a partial penetration of these markers in commercial markets as well

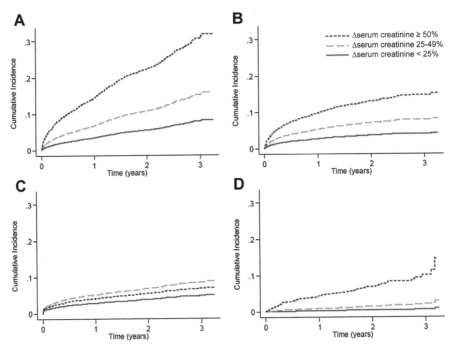

Fig. 1. Risk of mortality (*A*), heart failure (*B*), myocardial infarction (*C*), and end-stage renal disease (*D*) in patients undergoing coronary angiography. (*Adapted from* James MT, Ghali WA, Knudtson ML, et al, Alberta Provincial Project for Outcome Assessment in Coronary Heart Disease (APPROACH) Investigators. Associations between acute kidney injury and cardiovascular and renal outcomes after coronary angiography. Circulation 2011;123(4):411.)

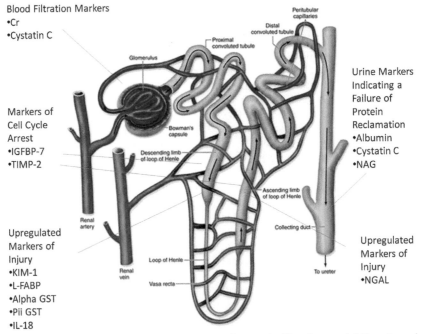

Fig. 2. Novel biomarkers indicating acute renal damage, reduction in filtration, and failure to reclaim normally resorbed proteins. Alpha GST, glutathione *S*-transferase α; Cr, creatinine; IGFBP-7, insulin-like growth factor–binding protein 7; IL-18, interleukin-18; KIM-1, kidney injury molecule 1; L-FABP, L-type fatty acid binding protein 1; NAG, *N*-acetyl-β-ᴅ-glucosaminidase; NGAL, neutrophil gelatinase–associated lipocalin; pii GST, glutathione *S*-transferase π; TIMP-2, tissue inhibitor of metalloproteinases 2.

as in prospective studies and clinical trials.[17] It is relatively clear, and similar to cardiac biomarkers of injury and their advancement from lactate dehydrogenase isoenzymes to creatinine kinase to troponin, that renal markers of injury will advance from less sensitive and specific (eg, serum Cr) to those that are able to detect AKI without a discernible change in eGFR. Just as troponin can increase in the setting of acute MI without a decrease in left ventricular ejection fraction, novel markers of CI-AKI elevate in response to injury with no change in serum Cr and, consequently, no decline in eGFR.[18] The authors have for many years used serum cystatin C as a companion filtration marker to serum Cr, which can be used in the detection of CI-AKI. Unlike serum Cr, cystatin C does not depend on muscle mass and tends to have a more rapid increase in blood concentration in response to injury. However, given that cystatin C is another filtration marker requiring a significant decrease in functional nephron mass to detect renal damage, it offers relatively little advantage over the more readily available serum Cr measurement. In Europe at present, both urine and serum neutrophil gelatinase–associated lipocalin (N-GAL, siderocalin-2) are available for the detection of AKI. The distal tubular cells produce large quantities of N-GAL in response to a variety of both acute and chronic injuries.[19] This protein works to limit the availabilities of unbound or catalytic iron released from the mitochondria of adjacent injured cells as a vestigial mechanism to reduce the bacterial growth of invading pathogens. Baseline N-GAL rises as eGFR is reduced, so there is no absolute cutoff for the detection of CI-AKI.[20] As a general rule, a doubling from baseline would indicate significant injury and be associated with adverse outcomes. L-type fatty acid binding protein is released by proximal tubular cells in response to many types of tissue damage. This marker is currently available as a urine test for the detection of AKI in Japan.[21] The most recent addition to the commercial market for novel biomarkers is the NephroCheck test, which is the mathematical product of 2 cell-cycle arrest markers released by proximal and distal tubular cells into urine: insulin-like growth factor–binding protein 7 (IGFBP-7) and tissue inhibitor of metalloproteinases 2 (TIMP-2).[22] The NephroCheck has been validated against standardized definitions of AKI in the intensive care unit, but has not undergone specific evaluation in CI-AKI.

How should these novel biomarkers be used in the risk prediction and detection of CI-AKI? To answer this question there will need to be specific studies in CI-AKI to understand the time course of the increase in blood and urine in relationship to the baseline. Because all of these markers are elevated in CKD, one must evaluate the peak to baseline ratio or an increase of 1, 2, 3, 5, or 10 times, similar to that of liver transaminases. The major advantages of these markers coming into clinical use in addition to serum creatine include: (1) they identify renal injury not detectable by serum Cr; (2) they increase much earlier (hours) than serum Cr; (3) baseline levels are elevated, hence the baseline levels can be used in conjunction with eGFR in risk prediction; (4) novel markers are independently and complementary to KDIGO-defined CI-AKI in the prediction of SAEs, including the need for renal replacement therapy and death.[17]

SUMMARY

CI-AKI is a well-studied complication of the administration of iodinated contrast. From baseline eGFR and diabetes as major risk determinants, and with higher contrast volumes or with more complicated procedures with hemodynamic instability, it can be anticipated that its occurrence can be as high as 50%. Probably as a marker of general frailty, CI-AKI has been associated with most major SAEs after PCI and, thus, has been of interest as a preventable complication in the catheterization laboratory. Novel blood and urine biomarkers will add considerably to the understanding of CI-AKI, and will undoubtedly expand the umbrella of concern regarding renal injury among patients undergoing PCI.

REFERENCES

1. KDIGO clinical practice guideline for acute kidney injury. Kidney Int 2012;2(Suppl 1):8–9.
2. McCullough PA, Adam A, Becker CR, et al. Contrast-Induced Nephropathy (CIN) Consensus Working Panel. Am J Cardiol 2006;98(6S1):5K–13K.
3. McCullough PA, Stacul F, Davidson C, et al. Contrast-Induced Nephropathy (CIN) Consensus Working Panel. Am J Cardiol 2006;98(6S1):2–4.
4. Guitterez N, Diaz A, Timmis GC, et al. Determinants of serum creatinine trajectory in acute contrast nephropathy. J Interv Cardiol 2002;15(5):349–54.
5. Li S, Chen SC, Shlipak M, et al. Low birth weight is associated with chronic kidney disease only in men. Kidney Int 2008;73(5):637–42.
6. Stolker JM, McCullough PA, Rao S, et al. Pre-procedural glucose levels and the risk for contrast-induced acute kidney injury in patients undergoing coronary angiography. J Am Coll Cardiol 2010; 55(14):1433–40.
7. McFarlane SI, McCullough PA, Sowers JR, et al, KEEP Steering Committee. Comparison of the CKD

epidemiology collaboration (CKD-EPI) and modification of diet in renal disease (MDRD) study equations: prevalence of and risk factors for diabetes mellitus in CKD in the Kidney Early Evaluation Program (KEEP). Am J Kidney Dis 2011;57(3 Suppl 2):S24–31.

8. McCullough PA, Brown JR. Effects of intra-arterial and intravenous iso-osmolar contrast medium (iodixanol) on the risk of contrast-induced acute kidney injury: a meta-analysis. Cardiorenal Med 2011;1(4): 220–34.

9. Laskey WK, Jenkins C, Selzer F, et al, NHLBI Dynamic Registry Investigators. Volume-to-creatinine clearance ratio: a pharmacokinetically based risk factor for prediction of early creatinine increase after percutaneous coronary intervention. J Am Coll Cardiol 2007;50(7):584–90.

10. Lele S, Shah S, McCullough PA, et al. Serum catalytic iron as a novel biomarker of vascular injury in acute coronary syndromes. EuroIntervention 2009; 5(3):336–42.

11. Akrawinthawong K, Shaw MK, Kachner J, et al. Urine catalytic iron and neutrophil gelatinase-associated lipocalin as companion early markers of acute kidney injury after cardiac surgery: a prospective pilot study. Cardiorenal Med 2013;3(1):7–16.

12. James MT, Samuel SM, Manning MA, et al. Contrast-induced acute kidney injury and risk of adverse clinical outcomes after coronary angiography: a systematic review and meta-analysis. Circ Cardiovasc Interv 2013;6(1):37–43.

13. McCullough PA. Contrast-induced acute kidney injury. J Am Coll Cardiol 2008;51(15):1419–28.

14. James MT, Ghali WA, Knudtson ML, et al, Alberta Provincial Project for Outcome Assessment in Coronary Heart Disease (APPROACH) Investigators.

Associations between acute kidney injury and cardiovascular and renal outcomes after coronary angiography. Circulation 2011;123(4):409–16.

15. Solomon RJ, Mehran R, Natarajan MK, et al. Contrast-induced nephropathy and long-term adverse events: cause and effect? Clin J Am Soc Nephrol 2009;4(7):1162–9.

16. McCullough PA. Cardiorenal syndromes: pathophysiology to prevention. Int J Nephrol 2010;2010: 762590.

17. McCullough PA, Bouchard J, Waikar SS, et al. Implementation of novel biomarkers in the diagnosis, prognosis, and management of acute kidney injury: executive summary from the tenth consensus conference of the Acute Dialysis Quality Initiative (ADQI). Contrib Nephrol 2013;182:5–12.

18. Ronco C, McCullough PA, Chawla LS. Kidney attack versus heart attack: evolution of classification and diagnostic criteria. Lancet 2013;382(9896):939–40.

19. McCullough PA, El-Ghoroury M, Yamasaki H. Early detection of acute kidney injury with neutrophil gelatinase-associated lipocalin. J Am Coll Cardiol 2011;57(17):1762–4.

20. McCullough PA, Williams FJ, Stivers DN, et al. Neutrophil gelatinase-associated lipocalin: a novel marker of contrast nephropathy risk. Am J Nephrol 2012;35(6):509–14.

21. Doi K, Noiri E, Maeda-Mamiya R, et al. Urinary L-type fatty acid-binding protein as a new biomarker of sepsis complicated with acute kidney injury. Crit Care Med 2010;38(10):2037–42.

22. Kashani K, Al-Khafaji A, Ardiles T, et al. Discovery and validation of cell cycle arrest biomarkers in human acute kidney injury. Crit Care 2013; 17(1):R25.

Pathophysiology of Contrast-Induced Acute Kidney Injury

Remy W.F. Geenen, MD[a],*, Hylke Jan Kingma, PharmD[b],
Aart J. van der Molen, MD[c]

KEYWORDS

- Contrast media adverse effects • Contrast media toxicity • Contrast-induced nephropathy
- Contrast-induced acute kidney injury

KEY POINTS

- Ten percent of the renal blood flow represents medullary flow.
- Po_2 levels of the medulla can be as low as 20 mm Hg.
- Blood supply to the medulla is derived from the efferent arterioles, which give rise to the descending vasa recta (DVR) at the corticomedullary junction.
- Contrast media (CM) cause medullary hypoxia by hemodynamic effects, an increase in oxygen free radicals, and direct CM molecule tubular cell toxicity.
- Points of action for CM to cause vasoconstriction seem to be the afferent arterioles and the DVR.
- Both medullary ischemia and tubular cell toxicity lead to increased formation of oxygen free radicals.
- Increased formation of oxygen free radicals leads to increased ischemia and cell toxicity.
- Therefore, the 3 pathways of contrast-induced acute kidney injury enhance and support each other.

INTRODUCTION

Contrast-induced acute kidney injury (CI-AKI) refers to acute kidney injury (AKI) after intravenous or intra-arterial administration of contrast media (CM). The 2 key mechanisms related to AKI are acute tubular necrosis and prerenal azotemia, that is, increased serum creatinine and urea resulting from kidney hypoperfusion.[1] The pathophysiology of AKI in general is complex, and most of the understanding of this condition comes from animal studies. Modern frameworks show that AKI has 3 major pathways: hemodynamic injury, systemic inflammation, and toxic injury.[1] Among the potentially nephrotoxic drugs, CM are

prominent.[1] In the pathophysiology of CI-AKI, 3 major distinct, but potentially interacting pathways are recognized: hemodynamic effects, increase in oxygen free radicals, and direct CM molecule tubular cell toxicity.[2] This article reviews the pathophysiology of CI-AKI by describing and explaining these pathways.

DIRECT CM MOLECULE TUBULAR CELL TOXICITY

Of the 3 pathways, the contribution of direct tubular cell toxicity caused by CM is the least understood. All types of CM, high-osmolar, low-osmolar, and iso-osmolar, display toxicity in

The authors have nothing to disclose.
[a] Department of Radiology, Medisch Centrum Alkmaar, Wilhelminalaan 12, Alkmaar 1815 JD, Netherlands;
[b] Department of Clinical Pharmacy, Stichting Apotheek der Haarlemse Ziekenhuizen, Boerhavelaan 24, Haarlem 2035 RC, Netherlands; [c] Department of Radiology, Leiden University Medical Center, Albinusdreef 2, Leiden 2333 ZA, Netherlands
* Corresponding author.
E-mail address: r.w.f.geenen@mca.nl

interventional.theclinics.com

in vitro studies of tubular cell cultures.[3] What exactly happens when CM come into contact with renal tubular cells in vivo is unknown. In general, the toxic effects of high-osmolar CM are more pronounced than the effects of low-osmolar or iso-osmolar CM, but all types of CM have negative effects on cell cultures.[3,4] Many toxic effects of CM on renal cell cultures have been described: apoptosis, redistribution of membrane proteins, reduction of extracellular Ca^{2+}, DNA fragmentation, disruption of intercellular junctions, reduced cell proliferation, and altered mitochondrial function.[3,4] Apoptosis especially has been associated with increased levels of oxygen free radicals,[3] underlining how cell toxicity and formation of oxygen free radicals enhance each other. Furthermore, iodine is well known for its cytotoxic effect on bacteria, but is also toxic to human cells.[4] To what degree the small amount of free iodine in CM solutions is responsible for tubular cell toxicity remains unknown.

OXYGEN FREE RADICALS

Oxygen free radicals are molecules that contain 1 or more unpaired electrons, such as superoxide (O_2^-) and hydroxyl radical (OH^-).[2,5] During successive reduction reactions, these highly reactive molecules are turned into water.[2] Less aggressively reacting molecules, such as H_2O_2, are called reactive oxygen species (ROS).[2,5] In the pathophysiology of CI-AKI these types of molecules play a key role, as they interact with the other 2 pathways. Once formed during hypoxia and/or cellular injury and exceeding the cellular scavenging capacities, they lead to a specific type of injury, the so-called ischemia/reperfusion injury.[6] This type of cellular injury is a combination of both hypoxia and oxidative damage.[6]

Hypoxia is due to alteration of the renal microcirculation induced by oxygen free radicals and ROS. The exact pathway by which these molecules act on renal vasoconstrictors and vasodilators is unknown, but oxygen free radicals and ROS trigger an increase in vasoconstriction induced by angiotensin II and endothelin I.[6] Furthermore, they reduce the bioavailability of the vasodilative nitric oxide (NO),[6] eventually leading to increased renal vasoconstriction. As CM administration already decreases medullary blood flow and increases the oxygen demand of renal tubular cells, this medullary ischemia is increased by the formation of oxygen free radicals and ROS. On the other hand, ischemia leads to increased formation of -oxygen free radicals and ROS, so both processes enhance each other.

Oxidative damage to cells is due to the oxidative stress of highly reactive molecules. Intracellularly an imbalance between oxidants and antioxidants occurs, in favor of the oxidants. This imbalance affects mitochondrial and nuclear DNA, membrane lipids, and cellular proteins.[6] The result is increased cell injury leading to increased formation of oxygen free radicals and ROS, creating a vicious cycle.

HEMODYNAMIC EFFECTS

Besides hemodynamic renal effects caused by cell toxicity and increased oxidative stress, CM also have a direct effect on the renal vasculature.

Under physiologic resting conditions, 25% of the cardiac output is directed toward the kidneys. The greater part of cardiac output is directed toward the cortex, to optimize glomerular filtration and reabsorption of water and salts.[7] The medullary blood flow is low; 10% of the renal blood flow represents medullary flow.[8] Its function is to preserve osmotic gradients and enhance urinary concentration.[7] Under physiologic circumstances, oxygen partial pressure (Po_2) levels of the renal cortex are approximately 50 mm Hg, whereas Po_2 levels of the renal medulla can be as low as 20 mm Hg (**Fig. 1**).[7,9] The most vulnerable part of hypoxic damage is the deeper portion of the outer medulla that contains the metabolically active thick ascending limbs of the loop of Henle. In this part of the tubular system, an osmotic gradient is generated by active reabsorption of sodium, a process that requires a relatively large amount of oxygen.[7]

Blood flow to the renal medulla is derived from efferent arterioles of juxtamedullary glomeruli. At the corticomedullary junction, these efferent arterioles give rise to the so-called descending vasa recta (DVR). These DVR gradually form a capillary bed that penetrates deep into the inner medulla. These capillaries eventually coalesce to form ascending vasa recta (AVR) (**Fig. 2**). The transformation from DVR to capillaries and thence to AVR occurs gradually, with accompanying histologic changes in the composition of the vessel wall.[10]

After intravascular administration, CM display a rapid distribution over intravascular and extracellular fluids. The distribution half-life is usually several minutes, ranging from 2 to 30 minutes. Only 1% to 3% is bound by plasma proteins.[11]

Metabolism of CM in the human body does not take place. CM are eliminated quickly through glomerular filtration by the kidneys. The elimination half-life, or time to clear half of the amount of CM in the blood, is approximately 1 to 2 hours.[11] In the

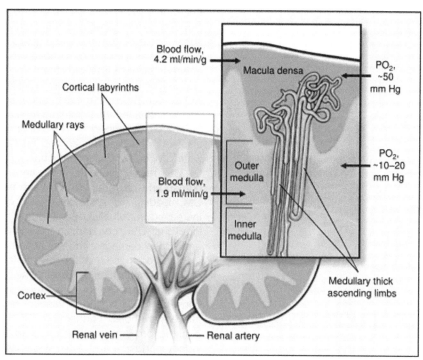

Fig. 1. Renal (patho)physiology. Po_2 of the cortex is approximately 50 mm Hg and declines to 25 mm Hg after contrast media (CM) administration. Po_2 of the medulla is approximately 20 mm Hg, and declines to 9 to 15 mm Hg after CM administration. The most vulnerable part for ischemia is the thick ascending limb from the loop of Henle in the outer medulla. (*From* Brezis M, Rosen S. Hypoxia of the renal medulla—its implications for disease. N Engl J Med 1995;332:648; with permission.)

first 24 hours after intravascular administration of CM, approximately 100% of the CM is excreted in the urine in patients with a normal renal function. In patients with decreased renal function the elimination half-life can increase to 40 hours or more.[11] Alternative routes of elimination, such as biliary elimination, are slow.

The hemodynamic response to intra-arterial injection of CM is biphasic: a brief initial increase in renal blood flow followed by a prolonged decline of 10% to 25% below baseline.[2,8,12] This process predominantly reflects a decline in cortical blood flow, as 10% of renal blood flow represents medullary flow.[8] Declines of outer medullary Po_2 by 50% to 67% after CM administration to 9 to 15 mm Hg have been reported.[5,8] The mechanism for medullary hypoxia is a combination of a decline in regional microcirculatory blood flow and the increased oxygen demand of tubular cells.[5,8]

Vasoactive mediators play a crucial role in the decline in regional blood flow after CM administration. Prominent medullary vasodilators include adenosine, dopamine, NO, atrial natriuretic peptide (ANP), and prostaglandin E_2.[7,9,12] Vasoconstrictors act more on the cortical vessels, to decrease glomerular filtration.[8] Potent vasoconstrictors include vasopressin, angiotensin II, and

endothelin.[7,9] Potential additional participants, with both dilative and constrictive properties, are serotonin, bradykinin, leukotrienes, histamine, and catecholamines.[12] It is unknown as to what extent each mediator plays a role in CI-AKI pathogenesis, but an imbalance occurs between vasoconstrictive and vasodilative mediators in favor of the vasoconstrictive mediators. Furthermore, the distribution of receptor mediator subtypes in the cortex and medulla may be responsible for different regional hemodynamic responses.[8,12]

Increased oxygen demand of tubular cells is a phenomenon that occurs after injection of CM with an osmolality higher than blood (ie, high-osmolar or low-osmolar CM). Injection of one of these types of CM leads to a transient increase in renal plasma flow, glomerular filtration, and urinary output, owing to their relative hyperosmolality in comparison with blood.[8] Because of both osmotic load and the effect of endothelin release, more sodium has to be reabsorbed by distal tubular cells,[5,8,9] which leads to increased oxygen consumption.[9,12] This effect is virtually nonexistent in iso-osmolar CM, a theoretical advantage of this type of CM. On the other hand, increased renal plasma flow, glomerular filtration, and urinary output, and a decrease in contact time between

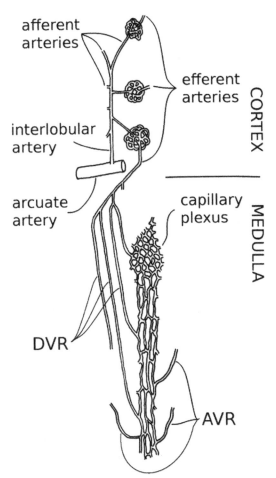

Fig. 2. Anatomy of the vascularization of the medulla. AVR, ascending vasa recta; DVR, descending vasa recta. (*From* Sendeski M, Patzak A, Pallone T, et al. Iodixanol, constriction of medullary descending vasa recta, and risk for contrast medium-induced nephropathy. Radiology 2009;251:699; with permission.)

the CM and renal tubular cells represent a theoretical advantage of high-osmolar and low-osmolar CM over iso-osmolar CM.

RECENT DEVELOPMENTS

In recent years, several animal studies have gained more insight into the pathophysiology of CI-AKI, especially the hemodynamic response of renal microvasculature on CM. Special interest has emerged in the response of DVR to CM. The average DVR diameter is 12 to 18 μm, close to that of a red blood cell. On isolated rat DVRs it was shown that microperfusion with iodixanol leads to a diameter reduction of 48%, caused by a decrease in NO production and an increase in reactivity of DVR to angiotensin II. Addition of a free radical scavenger prevented vasoconstriction induced by iodixanol and angiotensin II.[13] Additional research from the same group showed that iodixanol has a more pronounced vasoconstrictive effect on afferent arterioles than on efferent arterioles in isolated mouse kidney vessels. Decreased NO availability and increased superoxide concentration explained the increased tone and reactivity of afferent arterioles.[14] The same investigators also reported that human and rat DVR perfused with CM show vasoconstriction of 50.9% and 54.3%, respectively. In the same experiment, human and rat renal arteries were perfused with CM, leading to endothelial cell damage and increased endothelial permeability. It was postulated that DVR constriction is a consequence of endothelial damage and dysfunction.[15]

Based on these recent experiments on isolated perfused animal kidney vessels, one can postulate that the reduction in glomerular filtration rate caused by CM is due to vasoconstriction of the afferent arterioles. Furthermore, CM cause a DVR constriction. Both mechanisms lead to decreased kidney perfusion and, thus, decreased medullary perfusion. As these studies have been conducted with iodixanol as the agent investigated, it would be interesting to repeat these experiments with low-osmolar CM. The only additional study published in this area of research compared the effect on DVR constriction of the high-osmolar ionic CM amidotrizoate with the low-osmolar ioxaglate, the low-osmolar iopromide, and the iso-osmolar iodixanol.[16] All 4 types of CM showed DVR constriction rates between 45% and 63%. Amidotrizoate showed a constriction rate of 45% ± 7%, ioxaglate 53% ± 6%, iopromide 63% ± 11% and iodixanol 48% ± 8%. These differences were not statistically significant.[16] A recent publication has shown that continuous nitrite infusion improved renal tissue oxygenation by decreasing CM-induced vasoconstriction in rats.[17]

In general, iso-osmolar CM have a higher viscosity than low-osmolar CM, with comparable iodine concentrations. Recent results from animal studies suggest that compared with low-osmolar CM, iso-osmolar CM significantly increase urine viscosity, the expression of kidney injury markers, and the amount and period of time of iodine retention by the kidney. Furthermore, a decrease in renal blood oxygen levels and an increased formation of vacuoles in the renal tubular epithelium of the cortex, predominantly in the proximal and distal tubules, have been shown.[18,19] These animal results indicate that iso-osmolar nonionic CM have a relatively long contact time with renal tubular cells, leading to cell injury, which may be due to their relatively high viscosity.

SUMMARY

The passage of CM through the renal vascular bed leads to vasoconstriction. The perfusion decrease in the physiologically poorly oxygenated medulla leads to ischemia of tubular cells. Based on animal studies, the renal vascular points of CM action seem to be the afferent arterioles and DVR. Low-osmolar nonionic monomer CM increase diuresis and renal plasma flow by way of their relative hyperosmolality in comparison with blood. This process leads to an increased Na^+ supply and reabsorption in the thick ascending limb of the loop of Henle, which requires a relatively high amount of oxygen, thereby increasing the medullary ischemia. Iso-osmolar nonionic dimers have virtually no effect on Na^+ reabsorption rates, and therefore do not aggravate medullary ischemia by this pathway. Owing to the diuretic effect, animal studies show that low-osmolar nonionic monomers exert less tubular cell injury in comparison with iso-osmolar nonionic dimers. In the pathophysiology of CI-AKI, both types of frequently used CM have their theoretical advantages and disadvantages. Through both ischemia and direct toxicity to renal tubular cells ROS formation is increased, which enhances the effect of vasoconstrictive mediators and reduces the bioavailability of vasodilative mediators. Furthermore, ROS formation leads to oxidative damage to tubular cells. These 3 interacting pathways, namely hemodynamic effects, an increase in oxygen free radicals, and direct CM molecule tubular cell toxicity, finally leads to tubular necrosis.

REFERENCES

1. Bellomo R, Kellum JA, Ronco C. Acute kidney injury. Lancet 2012;380:756–66.
2. Katzberg RW. Contrast medium-induced nephrotoxicity; which pathway? Radiology 2005;235:752–5.
3. Haller C, Hizoh I. The cytotoxicity of iodinated radiocontrast agents on renal cells in vitro. Invest Radiol 2004;39:149–54.
4. Sendeski MM. Pathophysiology of renal tissue damage by iodinated contrast media. Clin Exp Pharmacol Physiol 2011;38:292–9.
5. Persson PB, Hansell P, Liss P. Pathophysiology of contrast medium-induced nephropathy. Kidney Int 2005;68:14–22.
6. Heyman SN, Rosen S, Khamaisi M, et al. Reactive oxygen species and the pathogenesis of radiocontrast-induced nephropathy. Invest Radiol 2010;45:188–95.
7. Brezis M, Rosen S. Hypoxia of the renal medulla—its implications for disease. N Engl J Med 1995;332:647–55.
8. Heyman SN, Rosen S, Rosenberger C. Renal parenchymal hypoxia, hypoxia adaptation and the pathogenesis of radiocontrast nephropathy. Clin J Am Soc Nephrol 2008;3:288–96.
9. Heyman SN, Reichman J, Brezis M. Pathophysiology of radiocontrast nephropathy. Invest Radiol 1999;34:685–91.
10. Pallone TL, Turner MR, Edwards A, et al. Countercurrent exchange in the renal medulla. Am J Physiol Regul Integr Comp Physiol 2003;284:R1153–75.
11. Speck U. Contrast media: overview, use and pharmaceutical aspects [corrected]. 4th edition. Berlin, Heidelberg (Germany), New York: Springer; 1999. p. 8–83.
12. Heyman SN, Rosenberger C, Rosen S. Regional alterations in renal hemodynamics and oxygenation: a role in contrast medium-induced nephropathy. Nephrol Dial Transplant 2005;20(Suppl 1):i6–11.
13. Sendeski M, Patzak A, Pallone T, et al. Iodixanol, constriction of medullary descending vasa recta, and risk for contrast medium-induced nephropathy. Radiology 2009;251:697–704.
14. Liu ZZ, Viegas VU, Perlewitx A, et al. Iodinated contrast media differentially affect afferent and efferent arteriolar tone and reactivity in mice: a possible explanation for reduced glomerular filtration rate. Radiology 2012;265:762–71.
15. Sendeski MM, Persson AB, Liu ZZ, et al. Iodinated contrast media cause endothelial damage leading to vasoconstriction of human and rat vasa recta. Am J Physiol Renal Physiol 2012;303:1592–8.
16. Sendeski M, Patzak A, Persson PB. Constriction of the vasa recta, the vessels supplying the area at risk for acute kidney injury, by four different iodinated contrast media, evaluating ionic, non-ionic, monomeric and dimeric agents. Invest Radiol 2010;45:453–7.
17. Seeliger E, Cantow K, Arakelyan K, et al. Low-dose nitrite alleviates early effects of an X-ray contrast medium on renal hemodynamics and oxygenation in rats. Invest Radiol 2014;49:70–7.
18. Lenhard DC, Pietsch HM, Sieber MA, et al. The osmolality of non-ionic, iodinated contrast agents as an important factor for renal safety. Invest Radiol 2012;47:503–10.
19. Lenhard DC, Frisk AL, Lengsfeld P, et al. The effect of iodinated contrast agent properties on renal kinetics and oxygenation. Invest Radiol 2013;48:175–82.

Predicting Contrast-induced Renal Complications in the Catheterization Laboratory

Judith Kooiman, MSc[a,b,]*, Hitinder S. Gurm, MD[c]

KEYWORDS

- Renal complications • Percutaneous coronary intervention • Catheterization lab

KEY POINTS

- Ten prediction tools have been developed for risk assessment of renal complications after percutaneous coronary intervention.
- The prediction tools contain more or less the same risk factors, although some scores use procedural characteristics to predict renal complications.
- As only 3 of 10 studies underwent external validation, there is a great need for further research on the already designed risk scores.
- Scores that are based only on preprocedural variables are generally preferable for clinical use, and the use of scores described by one of the following 3 authors, Brown, Freeman, or Gurm, is favored.

INTRODUCTION

The use of prediction rules or algorithms is increasing in daily practice of all types of medical specialties, the most famous probably being the Framingham risk model.[1] These prediction rules can aid physicians in their clinical decision-making by estimating the risk of disease or complications using patient characteristics that are readily available. Although risk prediction by algorithms or tools is not new, over the last decade the number of publications on prediction rules has increased remarkably.

This increased popularity of prediction rules is comprehensible. Directing preventive measures to an entire population at risk of a certain complication might not be feasible or advisable from a value-based care perspective. Risk scores or algorithms can therefore be very useful in targeting preventive measures to patients at high risk of complications, such as the need for new-onset dialysis after percutaneous coronary intervention (PCI).

Risk scores should undergo 3 analytical phases before they are suitable for adoption in clinical practice.[2] First, the risk score or algorithm should be derived from a study that clearly defined its endpoint of interest and that was conducted in a well-defined population; for instance, the risk of acute kidney injury (AKI) defined by the *Acute Kidney Injury Network (AKIN)* criteria in consecutive patients undergoing PCI. Preferably, within this study the prediction rule should be derived and validated in 2 different data sets. Second, external

The authors have nothing to disclose.

[a] Department of Thrombosis and Hemostasis, Leiden University Medical Center, Leiden, South Holland, The Netherlands; [b] Department of Nephrology, Leiden University Medical Center, Leiden, South Holland, The Netherlands; [c] Division of Cardiovascular Medicine, Department of Internal Medicine, Frankel Cardiovascular Center, University of Michigan Health System, University of Michigan Cardiovascular Center, 2A394, 1500 E. Medical Center Drive, Ann Arbor, MI 48109-5853, USA
* Corresponding author. Albinusdreef 2, PO box 9600, 2300 RC, Leiden, South Holland, The Netherlands.
E-mail address: j.kooiman@lumc.nl

validation should take place in several independent populations, for example, in other hospitals by different research groups. This validation is of importance because prediction rules tend to perform best in the population in which they were derived. Ideally, a third and final step should be considered in which it is analyzed whether targeting (preventative) treatment strategies to patients identified as high risk of the outcome of interest by the prediction rule improves clinical outcome. This step can be assessed by a so-called impact study.[3] Unfortunately, this step has rarely been applied to most prediction models in a rigorously designed study.

In this review, the most important risk factors are discussed for renal complications post-PCI, the prediction rules that are available in literature to assess a patient's risk of such complications, and whether these scores have been externally validated for their predictive value.

MAJOR RISK FACTORS FOR RENAL COMPLICATIONS POST-PCI
Pre-existing Chronic Kidney Disease

Patients with pre-existing chronic kidney disease (CKD) are at increased risk of developing AKI post-PCI.[4,5] The risk of AKI starts to increase below an estimated glomerular filtration rate (eGFR) of 70 mL/min.[6] The magnitude of this increased risk is directly associated with the severity of CKD and may be as high as 50% in patients with an eGFR 10 to 15 mL/min.

Pre-existing CKD is not only a risk factor for renal complications post-PCI but also has an impact on its clinical course. Patients with CKD are known to recover less frequently from episodes of AKI compared with patients without pre-existing CKD.[7] In a study of 1196 patients undergoing coronary angiography, 8 of 508 patients with pre-existing CKD (serum creatinine ≥1.5 mg/dL) had a need for new-onset dialysis due to AKI versus 0 of 688 in patients without CKD.[8] Moreover, Chen and colleagues[9] found increased 30-day and 6-month mortality in CKD patients developing AKI post-PCI compared with CKD patients in whom renal function remained stable and patients without pre-existing CKD that did develop AKI.

Diabetes Mellitus

Diabetes mellitus is a common comorbid condition in patients undergoing PCI, with about one-third of patients being diagnosed with this disease.[10,11] Patients with diabetes are at 2-fold increased risk of developing AKI post-PCI, regardless of the presence of CKD.[11–13] The pathophysiology behind this increased risk in patients with diabetes has recently been discussed in a review by Heyman and colleagues.[14] They concluded that the increased risk of contrast-induced AKI is associated with diabetes-induced alterations to the kidney that make it more vulnerable for hypoxic and oxidative stress induced by the contrast agent and impaired protective mechanisms aimed at the preservation of medullary oxygenation[14] in patients with diabetes.

High Contrast Dose

Iodinated contrast media can cause AKI, or contrast-induced nephropathy, via direct tubular toxicity and ischemic injury secondary to vasoconstriction at the level of the medulla.[15] Use of a high contrast dose at time of PCI increases the risks AKI and new-onset dialysis. Two formulas have been proposed to indicate the maximum contrast dose (MCD) above which the risk of AKI increases substantially. In 1989, Cigarroa and colleagues[16] proposed to calculate the MCD by (5 × body-weight [kg])/serum creatinine (mg/dL). This formula was later validated by external cohorts, among others by Marenzi and colleagues,[17] who found a 3-fold increased risk of AKI in patients receiving an MCD greater than 1.0. Although this definition of MCD has proven to be predictive of AKI post-PCI, it cannot be easily used as a rule of thumb in the catheterization laboratory. As a result, several research groups validated another definition of MCD, estimated by contrast volume (CV in mL)/calculated creatinine clearance (CCC in mL/min). The risk of renal complications post-PCI is markedly increased when the ratio of CV/CCC exceeds 2.0 or 3.0.[18,19] This simple formula allows for easy assessment of the MCD that could be used during PCI without increasing the risk of contrast-induced AKI.

Hemodynamic Instability

Contrast-induced nephropathy is frequently considered the only cause of AKI post-PCI. However, PCI is associated with several other causes of renal failure, such as hemodynamic instability indicated by cardiogenic shock, left ventricular ejection fraction less than 45%, or the use of an intra-aortic balloon pump before or during PCI. Depending on the definition, hemodynamic instability increases the risk of AKI by 3-fold to 15-fold. Hemodynamic instability can directly result in prerenal failure, causing an increase in serum creatinine post-PCI that cannot be distinguished from contrast-induced nephropathy. Furthermore, hemodynamic instability caused by hypovolemia activates volume preservation by renin-angiotensin system activation and vasopressin,[20,21] aggravating contrast media–induced medullary hypoperfusion. Following this, Ohno and colleagues[22] demonstrated AKI post-PCI to be associated with periprocedural bleeding, with the incidence of AKI correlated to the severity of the bleeding complications.

PREDICTION RULES FOR RENAL COMPLICATIONS POST-PCI

Since 1997, 10 prediction tools for renal complications post-PCI have been developed (**Table 1**). There is a considerable overlap between these scores in the risk factors that were included to assess the risk of renal complications. The 10 risk scores can roughly be divided into 2 groups. The first group contains only preprocedural patient characteristics and could therefore be used to assess the risk of renal complications before PCI is performed.[23–27] The second group of prediction rules contains among others procedural variables, such as contrast dose or time to reperfusion.[4,11–13,28] Consequently, these prediction tools are mainly useful for research purposes but cannot be used to target renal protective strategies to high-risk patients.

Prediction of Acute Kidney Injury Post-PCI

Seven of 10 prediction rules were developed to predict AKI,[4,11,13,24,26–28] of which 3 are solely based on preprocedural patient characteristics.[24,26,27] The definition of AKI post-PCI varies considerably between the different studies (increase in serum creatinine $\geq$0.5 mg/dL, $\geq$1.0 mg/dL, combination of $\geq$25% or $\geq$0.5 mg/dL), making it cumbersome to compare the performance of the risk scores. The predictive value of the scores as reported by the original studies varied widely, with c-statistics between 0.67 and 0.89. It should be noted that only prediction rules with a c-statistic greater than 0.80 are generally considered suitable for application in daily practice.[29] Therefore, based on the c-statistic reported by Mehran and colleagues[11] (0.67), their prediction tool would not meet these standards. This finding is remarkable because the Mehran risk tool is one of the most cited and validated prediction rules in literature on AKI post-PCI.

Prediction of New-Onset Dialysis Post-PCI

Three risk tools have been developed for the prediction of new-onset dialysis post-PCI,[12,25,26] of which one was also designed to predict AKI.[26] The risk score by McCullough and colleagues[12] contains a procedural risk factor (contrast dose) and cannot therefore be used to assess the risk of new-onset dialysis before PCI.[12] This score had a Hosmer-Lemeshow statistic of 6.82 (P = .45), indicating a good fit of the prediction model.[12] The predictive values of the scores by Freeman and colleagues[25] and Gurm and colleagues[26] were similar, with c-statistics of 0.89 and 0.88, respectively. Both scores solely contain baseline patient characteristics. As a result, they would both be suitable for preprocedural prediction of new-onset dialysis post-PCI, and therefore, for targeting preventative strategies to high-risk patients.

Brown and colleagues[23] designed a risk score for the combined endpoint of new-onset dialysis, or a serum creatinine increase of 50% or more or 2.0 mg/dL or more from baseline. This score does not include procedural risk factors and had a c-statistic of 0.84 in the internal validation cohort.

EXTERNAL VALIDATION AND COMPARISON OF THE DIFFERENT RISK SCORES

As mentioned in the introduction, external validation is an important step that should be taken before a risk tool can be implemented in clinical practice. Unfortunately, the number of risk scores for renal complications post-PCI that have undergone external validation is low. Only 3 of 10 scores have been tested in external cohorts by other research groups.

The score by Mehran and colleagues[28] is the most frequently validated risk score. Four studies validated this risk tool and found c-statistics ranging between 0.57 and 0.85.[30–32] A fifth validation study did not report a c-statistic, but demonstrated an increased risk of AKI in patients that were identified as (very) high risk of AKI post-PCI (odds ratio 4.6 and 4.9, respectively) compared with low-risk patients.[33]

The score by Bartholomew and colleagues[28] has been validated by 2 studies.[34] The predictive value of the score varied significantly between the 2 validation studies. Tziakas and colleagues[28] validated the Bartholomew score in patients undergoing elective or emergent PCI and defined AKI as a serum creatinine increase greater than 25% or greater than 0.5 mg/dL, while Bartholomew defined AKI as a serum creatinine increase greater than 1.0 mg/dL. Within the study performed by Tziakas, the Bartholomew risk score performed poorly, with a c-statistic of 0.59. The second study that validated the risk score by Bartholomew was performed by Skelding and colleagues.[34] Their definition of AKI was similar to that of Bartholomew. Within this validation study a c-statistic of 0.86 was reported for the prediction

Table 1
Prediction scores for renal complications after PCI

First Author	Population	Outcomes Predicted	Model Variables	Cut-Offs	Test Characteristics	External Validation	Performance in Validation Studies	On-line Risk Calculator
McCullough et al,[12] 1997	Patients undergoing coronary interventions (ie, balloon angioplasty, atherec-tomy or stenting) Validation set N = 1826 Derivation set N = 1869	New-onset dialysis	• eGFR • Diabetes mellitus • Contrast dose (mL)	NA	Hosmer-Lemeshow statistic 6.82, p 0.45	No	NA	NA
Freeman et al,[25] 2002	Patients undergoing PCI Derivation set N = 10,729 Validation set N = 5863	New-onset dialysis	• Peripheral artery disease • Diabetes mellitus • Preprocedural CKD (ie, serum creatinine >2 mg/dL) • Heart failure • Cardiogenic shock	NA	C-statistic 0.93 in derivation and 0.89 in validation set	No	NA	NA

Study	Population	Outcome	Risk factors	Risk categories	C-statistic	Externally validated	External validation results	URL
Mehran et al,[11] 2004	Patients undergoing PCI; Derivation set N = 5571; Validation set N = 2786	CIN (defined as ≥25% or ≥0.5 mg/dL serum creatinine increase)	• Hypotension • Heart failure • CKD (ie, serum creatinine >1.5 mg/dL or eGFR <60 mL/min) • Diabetes mellitus • Age >75 y • Anemia • IABP • CV	• Low risk <5 points • Moderate 6–10 points • High 11–15 points • Very high ≥16 points	C-statistic of 0.70 in the derivation set and 0.67 in the validation set	Yes[28,30-33]	• C-statistic 0.5732 • C-statistic 0.6830 • C-statistic 0.8531 • C-statistic 0.5928 • Odds ratio for CIN of 4.60 (95% CI 2.71–7.81) in high-risk and 4.89 (95% CI: 2.55–9.40) in very high-risk group, as compared with the low-risk group[33]	http://www.qxmd.com/calculate-online/nephrology/contrast-nephropathy-post-pci
Bartholomew et al,[13] 2004	Patients undergoing PCI; Derivation set N = 10,481; Validation set N = 9998	CIN (defined as ≥1.0 mg/dL serum creatinine increase)	• eGFR <60 mL/min • IABP • Urgent/emergent procedure • Diabetes mellitus • Heart failure • Hypertension • Peripheral artery disease • CV >260 mL	• Low risk <5 points • Moderate 5–6 points • High 7–8 points • Very high ≥9 points	C-statistic 0.89 in validation cohort	Yes[28,34]	• C-statistic 0.8634 • C-statistic 0.5828	NA
Marenzi et al,[4] 2004	208 patients undergoing primary PCI for STEMI	CIN (defined as ≥0.5 mg/dL serum creatinine increase)	• Age ≥75 y • Anterior AMI • Time to reperfusion ≥6 h • CV ≥300 mL • Use of IABP	NA	NA	Yes[32]	C-statistic 0.57[32]	NA

(continued on next page)

Table 1
Prediction scores for renal complications after PCI (continued)

First Author	Population	Outcomes Predicted	Model Variables	Cut-Offs	Test Characteristics	External Validation	Performance in Validation Studies	On-line Risk Calculator
Brown et al,[23] 2008	11,141 patients undergoing PCI	Serious renal dysfunction (defined as new-onset dialysis, or ≥50% or ≥2.0 mg/dL serum creatinine increase)	• Age ≥80 y • Female gender • Diabetes mellitus • Urgent PCI • Emergent PCI • Heart failure • Creatinine 1.3–1.9 mg/dL • Creatinine ≥2.0 mg/dL • Pre-PCI IAPB	NA	C-statistic 0.87 in derivation cohort and 0.84 in the validation cohort	No	NA	NA
Maioli et al,[27] 2010	Patients undergoing coronary angiography or PCI Derivation set N = 1218 Validation set N = 502	CIN (defined as ≥0.5 mg/dL serum creatinine increase)	• One procedure w/in past 72 h • LVEF ≤45% • Preprocedural serum creatinine ≥ baseline serum creatinine • Baseline serum creatinine ≥1.5 mg/dL • Diabetes mellitus • eGFR ≤44 mL/min • Age ≥73 y	• Low risk ≤3 points • Moderate risk 4–6 points • High risk 7–8 points • Very high risk ≥9 points	C-statistic 0.85 in derivation cohort and 0.82 in validation cohort	No	NA	NA
Tziakas et al,[28] 2013	Patients undergoing PCI Derivation set N = 488 Validation set N = 200	CIN (defined as ≥25% or ≥0.5 mg/dL serum creatinine increase)	• Pre-existing CKD[a] • Metformin use • Previous PCI • Peripheral artery disease • CV >300 mL	• Low risk ≤2 points • High risk >2 points	C-statistic 0.76 in derivation cohort and 0.86 in the validation cohort	No	NA	NA

Gurm et al,[26] 2013	Patients undergoing PCI Derivation set N = 40,001 Validation set N = 20,572	CIN (defined as ≥0.5 mg/dL serum creatinine increase) and new-onset dialysis	• Reduced model[b] • PCI indication • PCI status • CAD presentation • Cardiogenic shock • Heart failure • Pre-PCI LVEF • Diabetes mellitus • Age, y • Weight, kg • Height, cm • Creatine kinase-MB • Serum creatinine • Hemoglobin • Troponin I • Troponin T	NA	CIN C-statistic for reduced model in validation cohort of 0.84 New-onset dialysis C-statistic for reduced model in validation cohort of 0.88	No	NA	NA	https://bmc2.org/calculators/cin
Chen et al,[24] 2014	Patients undergoing PCI Derivation set N = 1500 Validation set N = 1000	CIN (defined as ≥25% or ≥0.5 mg/dL serum creatinine increase)	• Age ≥70 y • History of MI • Diabetes mellitus • Preprocedural hypotension • LVEF ≤45% • Anemia • eGFR <60 L/min • HDL <1 mmol/L • Urgent PCI	• Low risk ≤7 points • Moderate risk 8–12 points • High-risk 13–16 points • Very high risk ≥17 points	C-statistic of 0.82 in both the derivation and the validation cohort	No	NA	NA	NA

Abbreviations: AMI, acute myocardial infarction; CAD, coronary artery disease; CI, confidence interval; CIN, contrast induced nephropathy; IABP, intra-aortic balloon pump; LVEF, left ventricular ejection fraction; MI, myocardial infarction; NA, not applicable.

[a] Defined as previous admission for renal artery stenosis, acute renal failure, glomerulonephritis, obstruction, hematuria, nephrotic syndrome, or nephrectomy irrespective of baseline creatinine levels or glomerular filtration rate.

[b] Full model contained 46 baseline clinical variables and had similar predictive value.[26]

of AKI post-PCI, comparable with the c-statistic in the initial report by Bartholomew.

The third risk score that has undergone external validation is the score designed by Marenzi and colleagues that was validated in 2010 by Sgura and colleagues.[32] Marenzi and Sgura studied the prediction of AKI within the same population, namely, in patients undergoing primary PCI for ST elevation myocardial infarction (STEMI). However, their definition of AKI differed slightly. Marenzi defined AKI as an increase in serum creatinine greater than 0.5 mg/dL, whereas Sgura defined AKI as the combined endpoint of a serum creatinine increase of either greater than 0.5 mg/dL or greater than 25%. Marenzi and colleagues did not report a c-statistic for the risk score in their article but did demonstrate a significant gradation in AKI rates with increased points on the score. Sgura did report a c-statistic for the Marenzi score. Unfortunately, it was too low for use in clinical practice (c-statistic 0.57).

Only 2 studies compared different risk scores for AKI post-PCI within the same population.[28,32] Sgura concluded that the Marenzi and Mehran scores had similar but low accuracy in the prediction of AKI in STEMI patients, with c-statistics of 0.57 for both scores.[32] Tziakas compared the Mehran and Bartholomew risk scores and concluded both scores to perform poorly (c-statistics of 0.59 and 0.58, respectively). As mentioned above, the poor predictive value of the Bartholomew score might be explained by an inconsistency in definition for AKI. However, Tziakas and Mehran did use the same definition for AKI in their studies.

SUMMARY

Since 1997, 10 prediction tools have been developed for renal complications post-PCI. They contain more or less the same risk factors, although some scores use procedural characteristics to predict renal complications. Consequently, these later risk scores can not be used to target preventive measures to high-risk patients. In addition, because only 3 of 10 studies underwent external validation, there is a great need for further research on the already designed risk scores with a consistent definition of AKI post-PCI, preferably the AKIN criteria.[35] Until then, institutions should consider using one of the existing risk scores containing only preprocedural risk factors that fits best in their workflow. Because it is of importance to not only assess the risk of AKI but also that of new-onset dialysis post-PCI, it is suggested to use the scores by either Brown, Freeman, or Gurm.[23,25,26]

REFERENCES

1. Wilson PW, D'Agostino RB, Levy D, et al. Prediction of coronary heart disease using risk factor categories. Circulation 1998;97(18):1837–47.
2. Wasson JH, Sox HC, Neff RK, et al. Clinical prediction rules. Applications and methodological standards. N Engl J Med 1985;313(13):793–9.
3. Moons KG, Altman DG, Vergouwe Y, et al. Prognosis and prognostic research: application and impact of prognostic models in clinical practice. BMJ 2009;338:b606.
4. Marenzi G, Lauri G, Assanelli E, et al. Contrast-induced nephropathy in patients undergoing primary angioplasty for acute myocardial infarction. J Am Coll Cardiol 2004;44(9):1780–5.
5. Rihal CS, Textor SC, Grill DE, et al. Incidence and prognostic importance of acute renal failure after percutaneous coronary intervention. Circulation 2002;105(19):2259–64.
6. Ando G, Morabito G, de Gregorio C, et al. Age, glomerular filtration rate, ejection fraction, and the AGEF score predict contrast-induced nephropathy in patients with acute myocardial infarction undergoing primary percutaneous coronary intervention. Catheter Cardiovasc Interv 2013;82(6):878–85.
7. Hsu CY, Chertow GM, McCulloch CE, et al. Nonrecovery of kidney function and death after acute on chronic renal failure. Clin J Am Soc Nephrol 2009;4(5):891–8.
8. Rudnick MR, Goldfarb S, Wexler L, et al. Nephrotoxicity of ionic and nonionic contrast media in 1196 patients: a randomized trial. The Iohexol Cooperative Study. Kidney Int 1995;47(1):254–61.
9. Chen SL, Zhang J, Yei F, et al. Clinical outcomes of contrast-induced nephropathy in patients undergoing percutaneous coronary intervention: a prospective, multicenter, randomized study to analyze the effect of hydration and acetylcysteine. Int J Cardiol 2008;126(3):407–13.
10. Gurm HS, Smith D, Share D, et al. Impact of automated contrast injector systems on contrast use and contrast-associated complications in patients undergoing percutaneous coronary interventions. JACC Cardiovasc Interv 2013;6(4):399–405.
11. Mehran R, Aymong ED, Nikolsky E, et al. A simple risk score for prediction of contrast-induced nephropathy after percutaneous coronary intervention: development and initial validation. J Am Coll Cardiol 2004;44(7):1393–9.
12. McCullough PA, Wolyn R, Rocher LL, et al. Acute renal failure after coronary intervention: incidence, risk factors, and relationship to mortality. Am J Med 1997;103(5):368–75.
13. Bartholomew BA, Harjai KJ, Dukkipati S, et al. Impact of nephropathy after percutaneous coronary

intervention and a method for risk stratification. Am J Cardiol 2004;93(12):1515–9.

14. Heyman SN, Rosenberger C, Rosen S, et al. Why is diabetes mellitus a risk factor for contrast-induced nephropathy? Biomed Res Int 2013;2013:123589.

15. Seeliger E, Sendeski M, Rihal CS, et al. Contrast-induced kidney injury: mechanisms, risk factors, and prevention. Eur Heart J 2012;33(16):2007–15.

16. Cigarroa RG, Lange RA, Williams RH, et al. Dosing of contrast material to prevent contrast nephropathy in patients with renal disease. Am J Med 1989; 86(6 Pt 1):649–52.

17. Marenzi G, Assanelli E, Campodonico J, et al. Contrast volume during primary percutaneous coronary intervention and subsequent contrast-induced nephropathy and mortality. Ann Intern Med 2009; 150(3):170–7.

18. Gurm HS, Dixon SR, Smith DE, et al. Renal function-based contrast dosing to define safe limits of radiographic contrast media in patients undergoing percutaneous coronary interventions. J Am Coll Cardiol 2011;58(9):907–14.

19. Tan N, Liu Y, Chen JY, et al. Use of the contrast volume or grams of iodine-to-creatinine clearance ratio to predict mortality after percutaneous coronary intervention. Am Heart J 2013;165(4):600–8.

20. Seeliger E, Lunenburg T, Ladwig M, et al. Role of the renin-angiotensin-aldosterone system for control of arterial blood pressure following moderate deficit in total body sodium: balance studies in freely moving dogs. Clin Exp Pharmacol Physiol 2010;37(2): e43–51.

21. Reinhardt HW, Seeliger E. Toward an integrative concept of control of total body sodium. News Physiol Sci 2000;15:319–25.

22. Ohno Y, Maekawa Y, Miyata H, et al. Impact of peri-procedural bleeding on incidence of contrast-induced acute kidney injury in patients treated with percutaneous coronary intervention. J Am Coll Cardiol 2013;62(14):1260–6.

23. Brown JR, DeVries JT, Piper WD, et al. Serious renal dysfunction after percutaneous coronary interventions can be predicted. Am Heart J 2008;155(2):260–6.

24. Chen YL, Fu NK, Xu J, et al. A simple preprocedural score for risk of contrast-induced acute kidney injury after percutaneous coronary intervention. Catheter Cardiovasc Interv 2014;83(1):E8–16.

25. Freeman RV, O'Donnell M, Share D, et al. Nephropathy requiring dialysis after percutaneous coronary

intervention and the critical role of an adjusted contrast dose. Am J Cardiol 2002;90(10):1068–73.

26. Gurm HS, Seth M, Kooiman J, et al. A novel tool for reliable and accurate prediction of renal complications in patients undergoing percutaneous coronary intervention. J Am Coll Cardiol 2013;61(22):2242–8.

27. Maioli M, Toso A, Gallopin M, et al. Preprocedural score for risk of contrast-induced nephropathy in elective coronary angiography and intervention. J Cardiovasc Med (Hagerstown) 2010;11(6):444–9.

28. Tziakas D, Chalikias G, Stakos D, et al. Development of an easily applicable risk score model for contrast-induced nephropathy prediction after percutaneous coronary intervention: a novel approach tailored to current practice. Int J Cardiol 2013;163(1):46–55.

29. Ohman EM, Granger CB, Harrington RA, et al. Risk stratification and therapeutic decision making in acute coronary syndromes. JAMA 2000;284(7): 876–8.

30. Aykan AC, Gul I, Gokdeniz T, et al. Is coronary artery disease complexity valuable in the prediction of contrast induced nephropathy besides Mehran risk score, in patients with ST elevation myocardial infarction treated with primary percutaneous coronary intervention? Heart Lung Circ 2013;22(10):836–43.

31. Raposeiras-Roubin S, Abu-Assi E, Ocaranza-Sanchez R, et al. Dosing of iodinated contrast volume: a new simple algorithm to stratify the risk of contrast-induced nephropathy in patients with acute coronary syndrome: a new simple algorithm to stratify the risk of contrast-induced nephropathy in patients with acute coronary syndrome. Catheter Cardiovasc Interv 2013;82(6):888–97.

32. Sgura FA, Bertelli L, Monopoli D, et al. Mehran contrast-induced nephropathy risk score predicts short- and long-term clinical outcomes in patients with ST-elevation-myocardial infarction. Circ Cardiovasc Interv 2010;3(5):491–8.

33. Wi J, Ko YG, Shin DH, et al. Prediction of contrast-induced nephropathy with persistent renal dysfunction and adverse long-term outcomes in patients with acute myocardial infarction using the Mehran risk score. Clin Cardiol 2013;36(1):46–53.

34. Skelding KA, Best PJ, Bartholomew BA, et al. Validation of a predictive risk score for radiocontrast-induced nephropathy following percutaneous coronary intervention. J Invasive Cardiol 2007;19(5):229–33.

35. Section 4: contrast-induced AKI. Kidney Int Suppl 2012;2(1):69–88.

Biomarkers of Contrast-Induced Nephropathy
Which Ones and What Is Their Clinical Relevance?

Jolanta Malyszko, MD, PhD[a],*,
Hanna Bachorzewska-Gajewska, MD, PhD[b],
Slawomir Dobrzycki, MD, PhD[b]

KEYWORDS

- Contrast nephropathy • Biomarkers • NGAL • KIM-1 • Cystatin C • L-FABP • NAG

KEY POINTS

- Normal serum creatinine has several limitations as a marker for acute kidney injury (AKI), such as wide normal range; gender dependence; and effects of diet, muscle mass, muscle metabolism, drugs, and volume status.
- Biomarkers specific to the kidney can be viewed as belonging to 1 of 2 broad classes representing functional changes (eg, serum creatinine, serum cystatin C, urine output) or kidney damage (eg, proteinuria, urine and serum neutrophil gelatinase-associated lipocalin [NGAL], kidney injury molecule 1 [KIM-1], liver-type fatty acid binding protein [LFABP]).
- NGAL has several attractive traits, especially its rapid increase in response to kidney injury, typically within 2 to 4 hours. NGAL has clinched status as a promising biomarker for AKI.
- Knowledge about biomarkers has improved substantially, with NGAL being the most studied, followed by KIM-1 and then others.
- The search for "the troponin of the kidney" is far advanced; however, one should be aware that acceptance of troponin as a cardiac marker was also a long process.

However beautiful is the strategy, you should occasionally look at the results.
—Winston Churchill

INTRODUCTION

Biomarkers are biological measures of a biological state. A biomarker is defined as a characteristic that is objectively measured and evaluated as an indicator of normal biological processes, pathogenic processes, or pharmacological responses to a therapeutic intervention. Biomarkers are used to perform a clinical assessment, to monitor and predict health states in individuals or across populations so that appropriate therapeutic intervention can be planned. An ideal biomarker is safe and easy to measure, cost-efficient to follow up, modifiable with treatment, and consistent across gender and ethnic groups. Cardiologists use troponin daily as a biomarker of acute cardiac injury that serves to diagnose, stratify risk, and guide therapy. Therefore, a "troponin-like" biomarker of acute kidney injury (AKI) should be easily measured, unaffected by other biological

The authors have nothing to disclose.
[a] 2nd Department of Nephrology, Medical University, M. Sklodowska-Curie 24a, Bialystok 15-276, Poland;
[b] Department of Invasive Cardiology, Medical University, M. Sklodowska-Curie 24a, Bialystok 15-276, Poland
* Corresponding author.
E-mail address: jolmal@poczta.onet.pl

interventional.theclinics.com

factors, and capable of both early detection and risk stratification.

Radiocontrast Media

More than 70 million diagnostic radiographic examinations requiring radiocontrast media (RCM) are performed worldwide each year, with at least 10 million in the United States alone. Procedures using RCM include myelography, angiography (including cerebral arteriography), venography, urography, endoscopic retrograde cholangiopancreatography, arthrography, and computed tomography. Because of the progress in medicine and access to health care, millions of doses of intravascular contrast agents are being administered worldwide, to an increasingly elderly and vulnerable population, many of whom have preexisting chronic kidney disease (CKD) and diabetes mellitus, principal risk factors for contrast-induced nephropathy (CIN). This particular combination creates a "perfect storm" for increased risk and prevalence of CIN. In fact, there is no magical and safe volume of contrast agent to prevent the occurrence of CIN.

The administration of RCM can lead to a usually reversible form of acute renal failure (ie, CIN) that begins soon after the contrast is administered.[1] Most commonly CIN, or contrast-induced acute kidney injury (CI-AKI), is defined as an acute impairment of renal function as manifested by an absolute increase in serum creatinine of at least 0.5 mg/dL or by relative increase by at least 25% from the baseline value.[2] Serum creatinine peaks usually 3 to 5 days after RCM administration and returns to baseline (or a new baseline) within 1 to 3 weeks.[2] CIN is a nonoliguric form of AKI for most patients. In almost all cases, the impairment in renal function is mild and transient. In comparison with percutaneous coronary interventions (PCI), the risk of CIN is low following intravenous contrast administration, even in patients with CKD.[3] As a result of better access to health care, interventional cardiologists are being asked more frequently to perform PCI on increasing numbers of patients with several significant comorbidities such as CKD and/or diabetes mellitus. CIN is a potentially serious complication of PCI.[2] In addition, clinicians are now better informed about the consequences of even small changes in renal function; however, in most circumstances this has not translated into an improvement in the management of AKI, including CI-AKI.[4]

Markers of Kidney Injury

Traditional markers

For many years creatinine was the gold standard in the assessment of kidney function and estimation of glomerular filtration rate (GFR). "Normal" serum creatinine has several limitations, such as wide normal range, gender dependence, effects of diet, muscle mass, muscle metabolism, drugs, and volume status, In AKI creatinine levels stabilize within a few days. To date, the loss of kidney function in AKI has been most easily detected by measurement of serum creatinine, which is used to estimate the GFR. However, estimated GFR (eGFR) is of no use in determining kidney function during an acute insult, because up to 50% of kidney function may be lost before an increase in serum creatinine is detected. In addition, after RCM administration resulting in CIN, plasma creatinine concentration usually returns to baseline within 7 days, and less than 1% of patients go on to require chronic hemodialysis. Thus, current biomarkers of kidney injury, especially creatinine and protein in urine, are inadequate.

Creatinine is a poor biomarker for AKI, principally because of its inability to help diagnose the early phase of AKI, including CIN. In addition, creatinine is less accurate for patients with low muscle mass and unusual diets. Other challenges inherent in using creatinine as a marker for AKI, including CIN, may delay diagnosis and potentially misclassify the actual injury status.

Proteinuria is considered a sensitive marker of kidney injury and a means of determining recovery in addition to CKD and its progression. However, it is also not very specific; levels may rise with use of certain nonsteroidal anti-inflammatory medications, neoplasms, lupus, and rheumatoid arthritis.

In summary, neither of these traditional markers reveals the location of kidney injury. Other conventional biomarkers such as urinary casts and fractional sodium excretion have been found to be insensitive and nonspecific for the early detection of AKI. Similarly, other traditional biomarkers detected in urine, such as filtered low molecular weight proteins, tubular proteins, and enzymes, have also suffered from lack of specificity and standardized assays. Thus, different urinary and serum proteins have been intensively investigated as possible biomarkers for the early diagnosis of AKI. The window of opportunity is narrow in CIN, and time to introduce proper treatment after the initiating insult is limited, particularly when patients are discharged within 24 to 48 hours after the procedure. Therefore, there is an extensive ongoing search for potential early markers for AKI, especially in the upcoming setting of short-stay hospitalizations for coronary angiographies and interventions.

Potential early markers

There are several promising candidate biomarkers with the ability to detect an early and graded increase in tubular epithelial cell injury and to distinguish prerenal causes of AKI from acute tubular necrosis. However, there are certain actions to be taken before biomarkers can be used in clinical practice. Biomarkers should be validated in different settings of AKI (cardiac surgery, sepsis) and in different clinical centers; subsequently, rapid assays should be developed and tested. Finally, a panel of biomarkers should be developed, as it is unlikely that a single biomarker will suffice.

As urine sampling is considered noninvasive, the search for biomarkers focused at first on the urinary tubular enzymes and other low molecular weight proteins. Nowadays several urinary tubular enzymes are considered biomarkers of AKI/CIN, such as the following:

Proximal renal tubular epithelial antigen (HRTE-1)
α-Glutathione-S-transferase (α-GST)
π-Glutathione-S-transferase (π-GST)
γ-Glutamyltranspeptidase (γ-GT)
Alanine aminopeptidase (AAP)
Lactate dehydrogenase (LDH)
N-Acetyl-β-glucosaminidase (NAG)
Alkaline phosphatase (ALP)

Most of these markers are released from proximal tubular epithelial cells within 12 hours, which is 4 days earlier than a detectable increase in serum creatinine. However, no validated cutoff points currently exist to help distinguish prerenal causes of AKI from acute tubular necrosis.

Other urinary low molecular weight proteins are:

α1-Microglobulin (α1-M)
β2-Microglobulin (β2-M)
Retinol-binding protein (RBP)
Adenosine deaminase binding protein (ABP)
Urinary cystatin C

These proteins are synthesized at different sites, filtered at the glomerulus, then reabsorbed at the proximal tubule; they are not normally secreted into the kidney, so their appearance in urine reflects kidney damage. Although they are promising in prediction of AKI/CIN prognosis and in helping to distinguish prerenal disease from acute tubular necrosis, increased levels may be observed after reversible and mild dysfunction and may not necessarily be associated with persistent or irreversible damage. It should be stressed that the optimal method of reporting biomarker excretion has not been determined, and hinders comparisons between reported trials. In addition, urinary biomarker excretion may be reported as an absolute concentration, or normalized to creatinine excretion.

In general, biomarkers specific to the kidney can be viewed as belonging to 1 of 2 broad classes representing functional changes (eg, serum creatinine, serum cystatin C, urine output) or kidney damage (eg, proteinuria, urine and serum neutrophil gelatinase-associated lipocalin [NGAL], kidney injury molecule 1 [KIM-1], liver-type fatty acid binding protein [LFABP]). This review focuses first on the markers of kidney injury, followed by cystatin C as a marker of kidney function.

MARKERS OF KIDNEY INJURY
Neutrophil Gelatinase-Associated Lipocalin

NGAL was discovered during a "fishing expedition" with a cDNA microarray in which NGAL appeared as "the biggest fish," that is, the most upregulating gene in the kidney early after the ischemic or nephrotoxic AKI in an animal model.[5] NGAL is a protein, a member of the lipocalin family[6] (a group of molecules that bind low molecular weight ligands), and functions in various biological processes ranging from vitamin delivery to pheromone transport.[6–10] NGAL is expressed at a low level in human tissues including the kidney, prostate, and epithelia of the respiratory and alimentary tracts.[6] It is a monomer with a molecular weight of 25 kDa (polypeptide chain of 178 amino acids) with neutrophil gelatinase. It appears that this association is not functionally relevant.[11] However, because it associated with neutrophil gelatinase, NGAL is thought to be an acute-phase protein with upregulated expression in different inflammatory conditions and in different neoplasms.[12]

Recently it has been shown that NGAL binds small iron-carrying molecules, so-called siderophores, and is crucial in various states including bacterial infection and kidney injury.[10–13] Miethke and Skerra[10] suggested that iron-complexed norepinephrine directly served as an iron source for bacterial uptake systems, and that NGAL could function as an antagonist of this iron-acquisition process. Interestingly they also showed that a functional iron-uptake system was necessary for noradrenaline-mediated growth stimulation as well as its NGAL-dependent inhibition, and demonstrated for the first time that human NGAL not only neutralized pathogen-derived virulence factors but also could effectively scavenge an iron-chelate complex abundant in the host.

Because of its small molecular size (25 kDa) and resistance to degradation, NGAL is readily excreted and detected in urine. NGAL was found to be 1 of the 7 genes highly upregulated in the mouse model of ischemia-reperfusion injury.[4] NGAL accumulated significantly in the human kidney cortical tubules, blood, and urine after nephrotoxic and ischemic injury.[14] NGAL is synthesized systemically in response to kidney damage, filtered in the glomerulus, and then taken up by tubules; however, it may also be produced locally by injured tubules. Because of its low molecular weight, NGAL is freely filtered by the glomerulus. Kidney proximal tubules reabsorb NGAL by efficient megalin-dependent endocytosis.[15] As shown by Mori and colleagues,[16] systemic injection of labeled NGAL resulted in an accumulation of NGAL in the proximal tubules without concomitant appearance in urine. Thus, NGAL appears in urine after proximal tubular injury as a result of reduced NGAL reabsorption and/or enhanced de novo NGAL synthesis. In ischemic injury to the kidney, a model of AKI, NGAL was synthesized largely in the loop of Henle and collecting ducts, which are not the primary sites of ischemic renal injury.

The trafficking of NGAL in the setting of renal injury may be more complicated than was initially thought.[17] Schmitt-Ott and colleagues[15] assessed NGAL in the renal vein and found that it was somewhat locally synthesized and secreted into urine, rather than released into the circulation; they also suggested that urinary NGAL was derived at least partially from local synthesis in the kidney because of high fractional excretion of NGAL in the urine. On the other hand, NGAL protein, detectable in the postischemic kidney, was localized to the damaged proximal tubule in a lysosomal compartment. The investigators also hypothesized that although NGAL was synthesized in the distal nephron, it was delivered to the proximal tubule from the circulation.[15] This conjecture could be explained most likely by glomerular filtration of circulating NGAL and subsequent uptake by proximal tubular epithelia through endocytosis.[16]

Paragas and colleagues,[18] using an NGAL reporter mouse, demonstrated that the NGAL-Luc2-mC reporter responds to endogenous signals that illuminate sites of injury (NGAL expression) in vivo and in real time. In this elegant study they found that in ischemia-reperfusion injury, as evidenced by an increase in creatinine, the kidneys illuminate, indicating NGAL production at the site of injury. Following maneuvers that led to significant prerenal azotemia associated with hypernatremia, interestingly there was no NGAL illumination, indicating that prerenal kidney injury was not responsible for enhanced NGAL expression. Thus, NGAL may potentially be useful in differentiating prerenal kidney injury from acute tubular necrosis.[18]

In addition, it was reported that AKI resulted in a dramatic increase in NGAL mRNA in various organs, mainly the lungs and the liver.[19] Thus, NGAL could be released into circulation and present a systemic pool. NGAL could also come from activated neutrophils/macrophages or inflamed vasculature, frequently found in coronary artery disease, hypertension, and CKD.[20] Hemdahl and colleagues[21] reported that NGAL was expressed in atherosclerotic plaques, so might also be released into the circulation from inflamed/damaged endothelium in patients during acute coronary syndrome, PCI, or cardiopulmonary bypass.

In sum, NGAL is markedly upregulated and abundantly expressed in the kidney after renal ischemia. As shown by Mori and colleagues[16] by inducing reepithelialization and reducing apoptosis, NGAL may exert its protective properties, and may function to dampen toxicity and increase the normal proliferation of kidney tubule cells. In addition, by enhancing the delivery of iron, NGAL upregulates heme oxygenase 1, thereby helping to protect kidney tubule cells. NGAL has several attractive traits, especially its rapid increased response to AKI, typically within 2 to 4 hours. NGAL clinched status as a promising biomarker for AKI following a 2005 study at Cincinnati Children's Hospital Medical Center that showed it to be a sensitive, specific, and highly predictive early biomarker of AKI in 71 children undergoing cardiac surgery.[22] The cutoff value for 2 hours after cardiopulmonary bypass of plasma NGAL is 150 ng/mL with an area under the curve (AUC) of 0.96, sensitivity of 84%, and specificity of 94% for the prediction of AKI in the pediatric population. The cutoff value for 2 hours after cardiopulmonary bypass of urinary NGAL is 100 mg/mL with an AUC of 0.95, sensitivity of 82%, and specificity of 90% in predicting AKI.[22] However, a pediatric population undergoing any procedure with RCM is generally free of the comorbidities often found in adults, which might be reason for biased values for cutoffs in adults.

Initially NGAL was detected by Western-blot technique. The first commercially available enzyme-linked immunosorbent assay (ELISA) from BioPorto (Gentofte, Denmark) was an option. BioPorto's NGAL patent is WO2006066587. BioPorto has obtained the intellectual property rights for NGAL as a method for diagnosing AKI in several countries. The last patent application is under examination in the United States, as the US Food and Drug Administration (FDA) approval is awaiting evidence that information about NGAL concentration changes clinical care. Other companies also offer ELISA assays for NGAL, such as R&D Systems (Minneapolis, MN); however, the sensitivity of the R&D assay (0.04 ng/mL vs <2 pg/mL) is different from that of BioPorto, as is the assay range (0.156–10 ng/mL in serum, heparin plasma, saliva, cell culture supernates, urine vs

4–1000 ng/mL in urine, plasma, serum, tissue extracts, or culture media in ELISA NGAL assay or 25–5000 ng/mL with security range up to 40,000 ng/mL in The NGAL Test Reagent Kit RUO for Hitachi 917 analyzers).

Recently, the NGAL Test was designed to run on open channels of most chemistry analyzers, effectively giving almost any laboratory immediate access to a rapid and easy method to measure NGAL. Using just only a few drops of plasma or urine, the NGAL Test produces results in just 10 minutes and thus addresses the demand for urgent NGAL determination. Such NGAL assessment makes bedside diagnosis easy and noninvasive within a reasonable period of time. The NGAL Test is available for most popular analyzers. Applications in development are for Beckman Coulter AU5800 (Beckman Coulter, Brea, CA) and Ortho Clinical Vitros (Ortho Clinical Diagnostica, Raritan, NJ). Moreover, a standardized point-of-care Triage device (Inverness Inc, San Diego, CA) has been designed to measure plasma NGAL. Quantitative results are available in 15 minutes, requiring only a microliter sample,[23] which makes bedside testing feasible. Both plasma and urinary NGAL assessed by Western blotting correlated well with values obtained using research ELISA.[24]

Interleukin-18 (Interferon-γ–Inducing Factor)

Interleukin (IL)-18 is a proinflammatory cytokine involved in diverse functions including inflammation (innate immunity), ischemic tissue injury, and T-cell–mediated immunity.[25] It may also act as a neutrophilic attractant.[25] In 2004, Parikh and colleagues[26] demonstrated that patients with acute tubular necrosis had significantly higher median urinary IL-18 concentrations than those with other renal conditions (normal renal function, prerenal azotemia, urinary tract infection, and CKD). Therefore, they proposed it as a specific biomarker of proximal acute tubular necrosis. IL-18 was induced in the proximal tubule after AKI and was cleaved by caspase-1, and therefore appeared in the urine.[26] IL-18 is both a mediator and a biomarker of ischemic AKI as evidenced by increased expression of IL-18 in the kidney in AKI. Inhibition of IL-18 is protective against AKI in animal models, and IL-18 rises in urine of both humans and animals after AKI. In addition, Matsumoto and colleagues[27] found that urine IL-18 correlated with proteinuria and disease activity in patients with glomerulonephritis.

Kidney Injury Molecule 1

KIM-1 is a type-1 membrane protein with extracellular immunoglobulin and highly O-glycosylated mucin subdomain in addition to multiple N-glycosylation sites and a relatively short cytoplasmic tail.[28,29] KIM-1, a putative epithelial cell adhesion molecule (also known as Tim-1 [T-cell immunoglobulin and mucin-containing molecule]) is normally not detectable in urine and healthy kidney tissue, but is expressed at very high levels in proximal tubular epithelial cells soon after an ischemic or toxic injury.[30] It may also play a role in epithelial adhesion, growth, and differentiation.

KIM-1 is cleaved from the surface of damaged tubular cells and released into the urine by metalloproteinase. The ectodomain is shed, and can be measured in urine by immunoassay. This process is closely related to KIM-1 expression in renal tissue and urinary excretion. KIM-1 is one of the members of a family of related molecules with 3 members in humans, which are encoded by genes adjacent to the IL-4, IL-5, and IL-13 cluster on human chromosome 5q33.2.[29] KIM-1 is expressed predominantly on T-helper type 2 cells, and Tim-4, a natural ligand for Tim-1, is expressed on macrophages and dendritic cells.[31]

In the kidney, KIM-1/Tim-1 is a phosphatidylserine receptor that confers a phagocytic phenotype on epithelial cells.[32] This receptor is responsible for the uptake of apoptotic cells and exosomes.[33] Ichimura and colleagues[31] elegantly showed that KIM-1 is responsible for the clearance of debris from damaged kidney tubule. KIM-1 can be expressed and excreted in urine within 12 hours after the initial ischemic insult, before regeneration of the epithelium, and persists over time. Urinary KIM-1 was reported to be a noninvasive, rapid, sensitive, and reproducible biomarker of nephrotoxic and ischemic AKI in an animal model.

A rapid direct immunochromatographic lateral-flow 15-minute assay for detection of urinary KIM-1 (rat) or KIM-1 (human) has been developed.[34] Using this assay, more urinary KIM-1 was detected in the urine of patients with AKI than in the urine from healthy volunteers. The assay range was found to be linear, from 1 to 20 ng/mL (n = 4). According to Vaidya and colleagues[34] there was a significant correlation between the urinary KIM-1 band intensity using the rat KIM-1 dipstick and levels of KIM-1 as measured by a microbead-based assay, histopathologic damage, and immunohistochemical assessment of renal KIM-1 in a dose-dependent and time-dependent manner. The lower limit of detection was 0.5 ng/mL for rat RenaStick and 0.8 ng/mL for human RenaStick (n = 4).[34] The analytical recovery for rat and human KIM-1 was within the acceptable range, from 78% to 108% for 5 ng/mL and 75% to 106% for 1 ng/mL. A biomarker dipstick, such as for KIM-1, may thus provide sensitive and accurate detection of kidney injury in clinical trials and, eventually, in clinical practice. In addition, renal and urinary KIM-1 correlated with kidney damage and kidney function, but not with proteinuria in various renal disorders, as shown by van Timmeren and colleagues.[35] These investigators demonstrated that KIM-1 was associated with renal fibrosis and inflammation, as KIM-1 was primarily expressed at the luminal side of dedifferentiated proximal tubules in areas with fibrosis and in macrophages in areas of inflammation.

Liver-Type Fatty Acid Binding Proteins

Mammalian intracellular fatty acid binding proteins (FABP) are tissue specific: liver, intestinal, heart muscle, adipocyte, epidermal, ileal brain, myelin, and testis. FABP are members of the superfamily of lipid-binding proteins, which are expressed from a large multigene family and encode 14-kDa proteins. FABP serve as intracellular lipid chaperones, enabling the lipid transport to a specific component in the cell. Thus, FABP not only take part in fatty acid trafficking but also serve as early indicators of ischemic conditions. At present, their exact biological role and mechanism of action are far from being solved.[36]

L-FABP is a 14-kDa protein produced predominantly by the liver, its gene being located on chromosome 2p11 in humans. L-FABP is expressed in the hepatocytes and the crypt to villous tip of intestine from duodenum to colon. Owing to its small molecular weight it can be filtered freely through the glomerulus and is then reabsorbed in proximal tubule epithelial cells, partly by the megalin-dependent system. L-FABP is also expressed in the human kidney, predominantly in the proximal tubules in the nephron segment, which use fatty acid as a major source of energy metabolism.[37]

There are 2 types of FABP in renal tubule cells: liver type, L-FABP (FABP1) and heart muscle type, H-FABP (FABP3). Immunohistochemistry staining revealed that L-FABP and H-FABP are complementarily localized. L-FABP is found in the cytoplasmic region of the proximal tubules, whereas H-FABP is found in the cytoplasmic region of the distal tubules except for the macula densa.[38,39] Of note, the promoter region of L-FABP contains the binding site for hepatocyte nuclear factor, hypoxia-inducible factor 1 (HIF-1), and peroxisome proliferator-activated receptors (PPARs). HIF-1 controls the expression of the erythropoietin gene. It might be speculated that the mechanism of hypoxic regulation of L-FABP would turn out to be transcriptional, via the common oxygen-sensing regulatory pathway, and that L-FABP could serve as a marker of renal hypoxia. Renal tubule epithelial cells are rich in mitochondria and thereby are vulnerable under hypoxia. When peritubular capillary flow decreases it causes oxidative stress, leading to hypoxia and subsequent injury to the outer medullary region. Proximal tubules are more susceptible than distal tubules to hypoxia, and thus are more prone to injury. During hypoxia, such as during ischemia and reperfusion, proximal tubules became necrotic, whereas distal tubules become apoptotic. It has been shown that urinary excretion of urinary L-FABP reflects stress of proximal tubular epithelial cells and correlates with severity of ischemic tubular injury.[40]

Urinary N-Acetyl-β-Glucosaminidase

β-NAG is a lysosomal enzyme found mainly in proximal tubular cells and possibly in other areas of the nephron, and is a sensitive marker for proximal tubular injury of varying etiology.[41] Its relatively high molecular weight (>130 kDa) precludes filtration of the enzyme by glomeruli. The increase in urinary NAG activity indicates tubular cell injury, although it can also reflect increased lysosomal activity without cellular damage.[42,43] During the course of AKI, NAG levels remain persistently elevated in the urine. Urinary β-NAG peaks earlier than serum creatinine, namely after 1 day.[44] However, its discriminative power seems insufficient to allow clinical use for AKI diagnosis.[24]

Urinary Insulin-Like Growth Factor-Binding Protein 7 and Tissue Inhibitor of Metalloproteinases 2

Urinary insulin-like growth factor-binding protein 7 (IGFBP7) and tissue inhibitor of metalloproteinases 2 (TIMP-2) are both inducers of G1 cell-cycle arrest; they are expressed in epithelial cells and act in an autocrine and paracrine manner to arrest the cell cycle in AKI. Both sepsis-induced and ischemia-induced cell injury and repair are associated with cell-cycle regulation.[45,46] After sepsis or ischemic injury, renal tubular cells enter a brief period of cell-cycle arrest, presumably to prevent potentially damaged cells from dividing.[47] Both IGFBP7 and TIMP-2 were identified in a discovery study and were evaluated in the Sapphire validation study of more than 700 critically ill patients, and performed well in comparison with traditional biomarkers in patients with sepsis and postsurgery patients.[48]

Midkine

Midkine (MK; gene name, Mdk), a heparin-binding growth factor, regulates cell growth, cell survival, migration, and antiapoptotic activity in nephrogenesis and development. In addition, MK is involved in inflammation, as revealed by in vivo studies such as arterial restenosis,[49] rheumatoid arthritis, ischemic renal injury,[50] cisplatin-induced tubulointerstitial nephritis,[51] and diabetic nephropathy.[52,53] In the kidney, MK is expressed in both proximal tubular cells and distal tubular epithelial cells,[50] and to a lesser extent in endothelial cells,[54] and is induced by oxidative stress through the activation of hypoxia-inducible factor 1a.[55] In a preliminary study the authors found a significant increase in serum MK as early as after 2 hours when compared with the baseline values after PCI. It was also significantly higher 4 and 8 hours after PCI and returned to the baseline values after 24 hours. In addition, MK levels were significantly higher 2, 4, and 8 hours after PCI in patients with CIN.[56]

Hepcidin

The hepcidin gene is regulated by iron loading, hypoxia or inflammation,[57–59] and its protein is produced by liver and kidney cells.[60] Hepcidin is a peptide hormone that regulates iron homeostasis.[57] In a pilot study of a nested case-control cohort of 22 patients with AKI and 22 without AKI, Ho and colleagues[61] reported a greater postoperative signal-to-noise ratio for urine hepcidin levels in those patients who did not go on to develop AKI, suggesting that hepcidin may be the first clinically useful negative biomarker for AKI after cardiopulmonary bypass. In particular, the active form of hepcidin (hepcidin-25) may increase in the urine on the day after surgery in patients who do not develop AKI after cardiac surgery.[61]

In a few studies hepcidin appeared to represent an early, predictive biomarker of AKI in a model of ischemia/reperfusion injury.[62–64] In the study by Prowle and colleagues,[63] receiver-operator characteristic (ROC) analysis showed that lower 24-hour urine hepcidin concentration and urinary hepcidin/creatinine ratio were sensitive and specific predictors of AKI, with predictive accuracy similar to that of RIFLE criteria for AKI. This inverse association between urinary hepcidin and AKI after cardiac surgery may be a unique feature of hepcidin as a biomarker,[65] in comparison with more established biomarkers of such as NGAL, which are positively correlated with AKI.[66] In their pilot study the authors found a significant increase in serum hepcidin as early as after 4 hours after PCI in comparison with the baseline values. It was also significantly higher 8 and 24 hours after PCI. Serum hepcidin was significantly lower 8 and 24 hours after PCI in patients with CIN.[67]

Cystatin C, a Marker of Glomerular Filtration

Serum cystatin C has generated considerable enthusiasm in recent years as a marker of GFR. Cystatin C, a basic low molecular mass protein (13,359 Da), is produced at a constant rate by all nucleated cells. It is a polypeptide chain with 120 amino acid residues. Under normal circumstances, it is freely filtered by the glomeruli and totally reabsorbed in the proximal tubule, where it is catabolized.[68] In the absence of tubular dysfunction, its serum level reflects glomerular filtration and can be used as a functional marker for acute and chronic changes in GFR.[69]

Because it is not secreted by the renal tubules, as is the case for creatinine,[70] some limitation of creatinine (effects of muscle mass, diet, sex, tubular secretion) may not be a problem with cystatin C. Cystatin C may be more reliable than serum creatinine–based methods in estimating GFR, particularly in those individuals with a mild reduction in GFR, in whom changes in serum creatinine are typically not observed (the so-called creatinine blind range of GFR).[71] It has been reported that cystatin C increased faster than creatinine after a decrease in GFR, enabling earlier identification of AKI.[72,73] However, close scrutiny of reports in which cystatin C was compared with gold-standard markers has resulted in mixed reviews concerning its potential usefulness.[74] Unfortunately, levels of plasma cystatin C may also be influenced by several nonrenal factors including corticosteroid administration, thyroid dysfunction, systemic inflammation, neoplasia, age, and, eventually, muscular mass.[69,75] In addition, the lack of standardization in the measurement of cystatin C is an ongoing concern.

CONTRAST-INDUCED NEPHROPATHY AFTER PCI: STUDIES ON BIOMARKERS

In an invasive cardiology department, early detection of CIN would allow a predischarge selection of outpatients needing hospitalization for closer renal, metabolic, and volemic control. In addition, it may also allow introduction of preventive measures as soon as is possible. Therefore, several promising biomarkers of tubular insult have been under investigation to enable their validation and introduction into clinical practice.

In a recent study, Liebetrau and colleagues[76] reported that NGAL concentrations before PCI were significantly higher in patients with subsequent CI-AKI. However, there was no significant difference in NGAL concentrations 4 hours after PCI among patients with and without CI-AKI. The investigators also found that 1 day after PCI, urinary NGAL concentrations were significantly higher in patients developing CI-AKI, and concluded that urinary NGAL predicted CI-AKI when measured 1 day after PCI.

Similar findings in patients with CKD developing CIN after PCI were reported by Alharazy and colleagues,[77] who concluded that changes in serum NGAL and serum cystatin C from baseline at 24 hours (Δ values) were able to diagnose CIN 24 hours earlier than serum creatinine, with serum NGAL showing a superior performance. The authors measured urinary and serum NGAL before and 2, 4, 12, 24, and 48 hours after PCI. There was a significant increase in serum NGAL after 2 and 4 hours, and an increase in urinary NGAL after 4 and 12 hours after PCI. In multivariate analysis, the only predictors of serum NGAL 2 hours after PCI were serum creatinine, time of PCI, and hemoglobin A1c.[78] Next the authors looked at the effect of diabetes mellitus on biomarkers of AKI in low-risk patients (ie, serum creatinine within the normal range) undergoing PCI.[79] Serum NGAL was significantly higher in diabetic patients 2, 4, 8, and 24 hours after PCI, whereas urinary NGAL was significantly higher 4, 8, and 24 hours after PCI. In addition, NGAL levels were significantly higher in patients with CIN, starting at 2 hours (serum NGAL) or 4 hours (urinary NGAL). Even after 48 hours, serum and urinary NGAL were significantly higher in patients with CIN when compared with patients without CIN. Cystatin C was higher 8 and 24 hours after PCI in patients with CIN; IL-18 also followed this pattern, whereas L-FABP was significantly higher only 24 hours after the PCI. KIM-1 tended to be higher after 24 and 48 hours, but the difference did not reach statistical significance.[79]

These data corroborated with the findings of Shaker and colleagues,[80] who evaluated serum creatinine, NGAL, and cystatin C before, then 4 and 24 hours after coronary angiography and found a significant increase in serum NGAL 4 and 24 hours after coronary intervention relative to the baseline values. In a prospective study in patients with normal serum creatinine undergoing PCI for unstable angina, a significant increase in serum and urinary NGAL after 2 and 4 hours was found.[81] Urinary L-FABP showed the same changes, increasing significantly after 4 hours and remaining elevated up to 48 hours after PCI.

In the pediatric population, Hirsch and colleagues[82] reported a significant increase in NGAL in urine and plasma within 2 hours after RCM administration in 91 children with congenital heart disease who were undergoing elective cardiac catheterization and angiography with RCM administration. The AUC for urinary and plasma NGAL were excellent, with values of 0.92 and 0.91, respectively. However, patient demographics and RCM volume were not predictive of CIN. Diabetic children were also enrolled in this study, but the findings were in line with the authors' results.

In a study on patients undergoing coronary angiography using low-osmolar RCM, Ling and colleagues[83] collected urine samples for NGAL and IL-18 assessment before and 24 hours after coronary angiography. At 24 hours after the procedure, the urinary IL-18 and NGAL levels were significantly increased in the CIN group relative to the control group. The predictable time of AKI onset determined by IL-18 was 24 hours earlier than that determined by serum creatinine ($P<.01$).

Lacquaniti and colleagues[84] published an interesting study evaluating the utility of serum and urinary NGAL in depicting an event of CIN in patients who received RCM (iomeprol), gadoterate meglumine, or radiopharmaceutical technetium-99m. Significant changes were observed in serum creatinine and NGAL levels in the magnetic resonance imaging and renal scintigraphy groups; however, there were no cases of CIN in these groups, whereas in the iomeprol group an early increase in NGAL was demonstrated. Changes in serum creatinine level occurred 24 hours after iomeprol administration. On ROC analysis, NGAL showed excellent sensitivity and specificity (serum NGAL: AUC 0.995, 95% confidence interval [CI] 0.868–0.992; urinary NGAL: AUC 0.992, 95% CI 0.925–1.000) in predicting CIN 8 hours after iomeprol administration. Moreover, NGAL independently predicted CIN in the regression analysis. As reported recently, monitoring of urinary NGAL levels not only provides early detection of CI-AKI but also predicts the severity of CI-AKI in CKD patients undergoing elective coronary procedures.[85]

Rickli and colleagues[86] observed that the increase in cystatin C achieved a maximum at 24 hours after the application of the contrast agent. An early increase in cystatin C following renal injury was also reported in trials addressing renal RCM toxicity.[80,87] In CKD patients, an increase of greater than 10% in cystatin C 24 hours after PCI predicts CIN (as defined by a >0.3 mg/dL increase in serum creatinine), with sensitivity of 100% and specificity of 86% (N = 410).[88]

Bulent Gul and colleagues[89] studied urinary IL-18 values before, and 24 and 72 hours after PCI. IL-18 did not differ significantly between patients with CIN and controls; therefore, they concluded that their findings argued against the hypothesis that urinary IL-18 might be clinically useful as a biomarker of CIN. On the other hand,

24 hours after PCI, IL-18 levels were significantly increased in patients developing CIN compared with controls, reducing the diagnostic delay by 24 hours.[89]

Kato and colleagues[90] studied changes in creatinine, cystatin C, α- and β-microglobulins, NAG, and L-FABP in 87 patients with CKD undergoing elective catheterization with or without PCI. L-FABP increased on days 1 and 2 after the procedure in 31 Japanese patients with stage 3 CKD (ie, eGFR 30–60 mL/min), with a prevalence of CIN of 42%. There was also an increase in L-FABP 1 day after the procedure in 41 patients with stage 2 CKD (ie, eGFR 60–90 mL/min).

The authors found a significant increase in L-FABP 24 and 48 hours after PCI in both diabetic and nondiabetic patients, without any significant changes 2 to 8 hours after the procedure. Nakamura and colleagues[91] studied 66 patients with serum creatinine between 1.2 and 2.5 mg/dL, defining CIN as an increase in serum creatinine of more than 0.5 mg/dL or a relative increase of more than 25% at 2 to 5 days after the procedure. CIN was prevalent in almost 20% of the studied patients. The investigators also found an increase in urinary L-FABP levels the next day and 2 days after angiography in patients developing CIN. After 14 days serum creatinine returned to the baseline level, but urinary L-FABP level remained high. However, urinary L-FABP levels in the non-CIN group changed little throughout the experimental period.

Manabe and colleagues[92] studied 220 consecutive patients with a serum creatinine level of 1.2 mg/dL or higher who underwent elective catheterization. Serum creatinine and L-FABP levels were measured immediately before and 1 and 2 days after the procedure. CIN was defined as an increase in serum Cr level of 0.3 mg/dL or greater within 48 hours after the procedure. Urinary L-FABP levels were significantly higher in patients with CIN than in those without CIN before administration of contrast agent. ROC analysis showed that the baseline urinary L-FABP level had 82% sensitivity and 69% specificity, at a cutoff value of 24.5 µg/g creatinine. In the multivariate analysis, independent predictors of CIN development were L-FABP level of 24.5 µg/g Cr or higher and left ventricular ejection fraction of 40% or lower.

Ren and colleagues[44] demonstrated that in patients with CIN, urinary NAG and serum creatinine levels on days 1 and 2 were significantly higher than at baseline and in comparison with patients without CIN; mean levels were gradually returning to baseline by day 6. Compared with serum creatinine, urinary NAG levels peaked earlier in CIN

patients and increased much more. In addition, Duranay and colleagues[93] measured serum bone morphogenetic protein 7 (BMP-7) levels before and 48 hours after coronary angiography in patients with baseline serum creatinine of more than 1.4 mg/dL. Concentrations of serum BMP-7 significantly decreased in the CIN group in comparison with baseline (488.6 ± 56.8 vs 356.4 ± 24.8, $P = .01$), whereas the concentration of BMP-7 did not change in patients without CIN (444.6 ± 54.6 vs 440.0 ± 53.9, $P = .09$).

BIOMARKERS OF CIN: WHICH ONES, AND WHAT IS THEIR CLINICAL RELEVANCE?

In a recent review on the biomarkers of AKI it was stated that the use of biomarkers in CIN is also prone to problems.[94] From the 8 studies exploring the use of biomarkers in CIN included in this review, 7 different definitions of CIN were used, making valid comparison virtually impossible. The sample sizes for research ranged from 30 to 410 and event numbers from 2 to 34 patients. Areas under ROC curves presented were relatively good and varied from 0.73 to 0.93. Positive and negative predictive values ranged from 20% to 68% and from 96% to 100%, respectively. Kidney-specific biomarkers have seen very limited clinical application, despite availability for clinical use in several regions worldwide. It was stressed in most studies that kidney biomarkers appeared earlier than serum creatinine; proof that the specificity of biomarker changes to diagnose actual changes in renal pathology (the gold standard) has been lacking. Instead the current, functional AKI/CIN biomarkers (serum creatinine and urine-output changes) have served as the "bronze standard" for most studies focused on the validation of novel AKI biomarkers, only a few of which included kidney biopsy information.[95] However, it must be stressed that kidney biopsy is not a standard for the diagnosis of CIN; therefore, investigators need to think about the appropriate comparators in the validation study of CIN biomarkers. Biomarkers cannot be judged as being better than creatinine, based on creatinine alone; however, in the case of CIN case it seems that we have no other comparator apart from our old friend creatinine, with all its limitations. Unfortunately, very scarce data exist on the utility of incorporating these novel biomarkers with creatinine and urine-output data to enhance the clinical care of patients with CIN. Finally, one should take into account the real-life scenario: shorter stay in hospital; an aging population with significant comorbidities; general inability to perform urinary-output assessment on an everyday basis in invasive cardiology, as patients are admitted to catheterization laboratories at any time; and, in the case of primary angioplasty, the greater importance of timely intervention with PCI than consideration of urine output.

In clinical practice it is likely that urinary markers will be more sensitive for true histologic damage, whereas serum levels of markers will probably be more sensitive for clearance changes. Urinary markers are noninvasive and easy to obtain, but their levels need to be standardized with those of creatinine excretion. Point-of-care devices or other bedside tests to implement protective or therapeutic measures in a timely manner are required.

In the last decade, many articles have been published on the use of new urinary and serum biomarkers for AKI/CIN. Nevertheless, a gap remains between the fascinating findings at the basic science level and the clinical application of this knowledge. In addition, clinicians need to define what degree of subclinical damage as detected by biomarkers is deemed acceptable. Knowledge of biomarkers has improved substantially, with NGAL being the most studied, followed by KIM-1 and the others. There are still questions pending about the cutoff value, predictive value in regard of need for renal replacement therapy, progression to CKD, and mortality. Lastly, the cost-effectiveness of a new biomarker or panel of biomarkers needs to be proved before they are incorporated into daily clinical practice.

REFERENCES

1. Berns AS. Nephrotoxicity of contrast media. Kidney Int 1989;36:730–40.
2. Gami AS, Garovic VD. Contrast nephropathy after coronary angiography. Mayo Clin Proc 2004;79: 211–9.
3. Weisbord SD, Mor MK, Resnick AL, et al. Incidence and outcomes of contrast-induced AKI following computed tomography. Clin J Am Soc Nephrol 2008;3:1274–81.
4. Stewart JF, Smith N, Kelly K, et al. Adding insult to injury: a review of the care of patients who died in hospital with a primary diagnosis of acute kidney injury (acute renal failure). A report by the National Confidential Enquiry into Patient Outcome and Death. 2009. Available at: http://www.ncepod.org.uk/2009aki.htm. Accessed February 10, 2014.
5. Mishra J, Ma Q, Prada A, et al. Identification of neutrophil gelatinase-associated lipocalin as a novel early urinary biomarker for ischemic renal injury. J Am Soc Nephrol 2003;14:2534–43.
6. Kjeldsen L, Johnsen AH, Sengelov H, et al. Isolation and primary structure of NGAL, a novel protein associated with human neutrophil gelatinase. J Biol Chem 1993;268:10425–32.
7. Cowland JB, Borregaard N. Molecular characterization and pattern of tissue expression of the gene for neutrophil gelatinase-associated lipocalin from humans. Genomics 1997;45:17–23.
8. Borregaard N, Cowland JB. Neutrophil gelatinase-associated lipocalin, a siderophore-binding eukaryotic protein. Biometals 2006;19:211–5.
9. Tong Z, Wu X, Ovcharenko D, et al. Neutrophil gelatinase-associated lipocalin as a survival factor. Biochem J 2005;391:441–8.
10. Miethke M, Skerra A. Neutrophil gelatinase-associated lipocalin possesses antimicrobial activity by interfering with L-norepinephrine-mediated bacterial iron acquisition. Antimicrob Agents Chemother 2010;54:1580–9.
11. Goetz DH, Holmes MA, Borregaard N, et al. The neutrophil lipocalin NGAL is a bacteriostatic agent that interferes with siderophore-mediated iron acquisition. Mol Cell 2002;10:1033–43.
12. Yang J, Goetz D, Li JY, et al. An iron delivery pathway mediated by a lipocalin. Mol Cell 2002; 10:1045–56.
13. Yang J, Mori K, Li JY, et al. Iron, lipocalin, and kidney epithelia. Am J Physiol Renal Physiol 2003;285: F9–18.
14. Mishra J, Mori K, Ma Q, et al. Amelioration of ischemic acute renal injury by neutrophil gelatinase-associated lipocalin. J Am Soc Nephrol 2004;15:3073–82.
15. Schmitt-Ott KM, Mori K, Li JY, et al. Dual action of neutrophil gelatinase-associated lipocalin. J Am Soc Nephrol 2007;18:407–13.
16. Mori K, Lee HT, Rapoport D, et al. Endocytic delivery of lipocalin-siderophore-iron complex rescues the kidney from ischemia-reperfusion injury. J Clin Invest 2005;115:610–21.
17. Schmidt-Ott KM, Mori K, Kalandadze A, et al. Neutrophil gelatinase-associated lipocalin-mediated iron traffic in kidney epithelia. Curr Opin Nephrol Hypertens 2006;15:442–9.
18. Paragas N, Qiu A, Zhang Q, et al. The Ngal reporter mouse detects the response of the kidney to injury in real time. Nat Med 2011;17:216.
19. Grigoryev DN, Liu M, Hassoun HT. The local and systemic inflammatory transcriptome after acute kidney injury. J Am Soc Nephrol 2008; 19:547–58.
20. Okusa MD. The inflammatory cascade in acute ischemic renal failure. Nephron 2002;90:133–8.
21. Hemdahl AL, Gabrielsen A, Zhu C, et al. Expression of neutrophil gelatinase-associated lipocalin in atherosclerosis and myocardial infarction. Arterioscler Thromb Vasc Biol 2006;26:136–42.
22. Mishra J, Dent C, Tarabishi R, et al. Neutrophil gelatinase-associated lipocalin (NGAL) as a

biomarker for acute renal injury after cardiac surgery. Lancet 2005;365:1231–8.

23. Dent CL, Ma Q, Dastrala S, et al. Plasma NGAL predicts acute kidney injury, morbidity and mortality after pediatric cardiac surgery: a prospective uncontrolled cohort study. Crit Care 2007;11: R127.

24. Nickolas TL, O'Rourke MJ, Yang J, et al. Sensitivity and specificity of a single emergency department measurement of urinary neutrophil gelatinase-associated lipocalin for diagnosing acute kidney injury. Ann Intern Med 2008;148:810–9.

25. Melnikov VY, Ecder T, Fantuzzi G, et al. Impaired IL-18 processing protects caspase-1-deficient mice from ischemic acute renal failure. J Clin Invest 2001;107:1145–52.

26. Parikh CR, Jani A, Melnikov VY, et al. Urinary interleukin-18 is a marker of human acute tubular necrosis. Am J Kidney Dis 2004;43:405–14.

27. Matsumoto K, Kanmatsuse K. Elevated interleukin-18 levels in the urine of nephrotic patients. Nephron 2001;88:334–9.

28. Ichimura T, Bonventre JV, Bailly V, et al. Kidney injury molecule-1 (KIM-1), a putative epithelial cell adhesion molecule containing a novel immunoglobulin domain, is up-regulated in renal cells after injury. J Biol Chem 1998;273:4135–42.

29. Monney L, Sabatos CA, Gaglia JL, et al. Th1-specific cell surface protein Tim-3 regulates macrophage activation and severity of an autoimmune disease. Nature 2002;415:536–41.

30. Han WK, Bailly V, Abichandani R, et al. Kidney Injury Molecule-1 (KIM-1): a novel biomarker for human renal proximal tubule injury. Kidney Int 2002;62:237–44.

31. Ichimura T, Asseldonk EJ, Humphreys BD, et al. Kidney injury molecule-1 is a phosphatidylserine receptor that confers a phagocytic phenotype on epithelial cells. J Clin Invest 2008;118:1657–68.

32. Meyers JH, Chakravarti S, Schlesinger D, et al. TIM-4 is the ligand for TIM-1, and the TIM-1-TIM-4 interaction regulates T cell proliferation. Nat Immunol 2005;6:455–64.

33. Kobayashi N, Karisola P, Peña-Cruz V, et al. TIM-1 and TIM-4 glycoproteins bind phosphatidylserine and mediate uptake of apoptotic cells. Immunity 2007;27:927–40.

34. Vaidya VS, Ford GM, Waikar SS, et al. A rapid urine test for early detection of kidney injury. Kidney Int 2009;76:108.

35. van Timmeren MM, van den Heuvel MC, Bailly V, et al. Tubular kidney injury molecule-1 (KIM-1) in human renal disease. J Pathol 2007;212:209–17.

36. Furuhashi M, Hotamisligil GS. Fatty acid-binding proteins: role in metabolic diseases and potential as drug targets. Nat Rev Drug Discov 2008;7: 489–503.

37. Portilla D, Dent C, Sugaya T, et al. Liver fatty acid-binding protein as a biomarker of acute kidney injury after cardiac surgery. Kidney Int 2008;73:465–72.

38. Maatman RG, Van Kuppevelt TH, Veerkamp JH. Two types of fatty acid-binding protein in human kidney. Isolation, characterization and localization. Biochem J 1991;273:759–66.

39. Yamamoto T, Noiri E, Ono Y, et al. Renal L-type fatty acid–binding protein in acute ischemic injury. J Am Soc Nephrol 2007;18:2894–902.

40. Kamijo A, Sugaya T, Hikawa A, et al. Urinary excretion of fatty acid-binding protein reflects stress overload on the proximal tubules. Am J Pathol 2004;165:1243.

41. Han WK, Waikar SS, Johnson A, et al. Urinary biomarkers in the early diagnosis of acute kidney injury. Kidney Int 2008;73:863–9.

42. Trof RJ, Di Maggio F, Leemreis J, et al. Biomarkers of acute renal injury and renal failure. Shock 2006; 26:245–53.

43. Liangos O, Perianayagam MC, Vaidya VS, et al. Urinary N-acetyl-β-(D)-glucosaminidase activity and kidney injury molecule-1 level are associated with adverse outcomes in acute renal failure. J Am Soc Nephrol 2007;18:904–12.

44. Ren L, Ji J, Fang Y, et al. Assessment of urinary N-acetyl-β-glucosaminidase as an early marker of contrast-induced nephropathy. J Int Med Res 2011;39:647–53.

45. Witzgall R, Brown D, Schwarz C, et al. Localization of proliferating cell nuclear antigen, vimentin, c-Fos, and clusterin in the postischemic kidney. Evidence for a heterogenous genetic response among nephron segments, and a large pool of mitotically active and dedifferentiated cells. J Clin Invest 1994;93:2175.

46. Yang QH, Liu DW, Long Y, et al. Acute renal failure during sepsis: potential role of cell cycle regulation. J Infect 2009;58:459.

47. Yang L, Besschetnova TY, Brooks CR, et al. Epithelial cell cycle arrest in G2/M mediates kidney fibrosis after injury. Nat Med 2010;16:535–43.

48. Kashani K, Al-Khafaji A, Ardiles T, et al. Discovery and validation of cell cycle arrest biomarkers in human acute kidney injury. Crit Care 2013;17:R25.

49. Horiba M, Kadomatsu K, Nakamura E, et al. Neointima formation in a restenosis model is suppressed in midkine-deficient mice. J Clin Invest 2000;105: 489–95.

50. Sato W, Kadomatsu K, Yuzawa Y, et al. Midkine is involved in neutrophil infiltration into the tubulointerstitium in ischemic renal injury. J Immunol 2001; 167:3463–9.

51. Kawai H, Sato W, Yuzawa Y, et al. Lack of the growth factor midkine enhances survival against cisplatin-induced renal damage. Am J Pathol 2004;165:1603–12.

52. Kosugi T, Yuzawa Y, Sato W, et al. Midkine is involved in tubulointerstitial inflammation associated with diabetic nephropathy. Lab Invest 2007; 87:903–13.

53. Kosugi T, Yuzawa Y, Sato W, et al. Growth factor midkine is involved in the pathogenesis of diabetic nephropathy. Am J Pathol 2006;168:9–19.

54. Kato K, Kosugi T, Sato W, et al. Growth factor Midkine is involved in the pathogenesis of renal injury induced by protein overload containing endotoxin. Clin Exp Nephrol 2011;15:346–54.

55. Reynolds PR, Mucenski ML, Le Cras TD, et al. Midkine is regulated by hypoxia and causes pulmonary vascular remodeling. J Biol Chem 2004;279: 37124–32.

56. Malyszko J, Malyszko JS, Gajewska H, et al. Midkine- possible novel biomarker of CI-AKI in patients undergoing PCI. J Am Soc Nephrol 2013;24:637A.

57. Ganz T. Molecular control of iron transport. J Am Soc Nephrol 2007;18:394–400.

58. Pigeon C, Ilyin G, Courselaud B, et al. A new mouse liver-specific gene, encoding a protein homologous to human antimicrobial peptide hepcidin, is overexpressed during iron overload. J Biol Chem 2001;276:7811–9.

59. Hunter HN, Fulton DB, Ganz T, et al. The solution structure of human hepcidin, a peptide hormone with antimicrobial activity that is involved in iron uptake and hereditary hemochromatosis. J Biol Chem 2002;277:37597–603.

60. Kulaksiz H, Theilig F, Bachmann S, et al. The iron-regulatory peptide hormone hepcidin: expression and cellular localization in the mammalian kidney. J Endocrinol 2005;184:361–70.

61. Ho J, Lucy M, Krokhin O, et al. Mass spectrometry-based proteomic analysis of urine in acute kidney injury following cardiopulmonary bypass: a nested case-control study. Am J Kidney Dis 2009;53: 584–95.

62. Haase-Fielitz A, Mertens PR, Plass M, et al. Urine hepcidin has additive value in ruling out cardiopulmonary bypass-associated acute kidney injury: an observational cohort study. Crit Care 2011;15: R186.

63. Prowle JR, Ostland V, Calzavacca P, et al. Greater increase in urinary hepcidin predicts protection from acute kidney injury after cardiopulmonary bypass. Nephrol Dial Transplant 2012;27:595–602.

64. Ho J, Reslerova M, Gali B, et al. Urinary hepcidin-25 and risk of acute kidney injury following cardiopulmonary bypass. Clin J Am Soc Nephrol 2011;6: 2340–6.

65. Haase M, Bellomo R, Haase-Fielitz A. Novel biomarkers, oxidative stress, and the role of labile iron toxicity in cardiopulmonary bypass associated acute kidney injury. J Am Coll Cardiol 2010;55: 2024–33.

66. Prowle JR, Westerman M, Bellomo R. Urinary hepcidin: an inverse biomarker of acute kidney injury after cardiopulmonary bypass? Curr Opin Crit Care 2010;16:540–4.

67. Malyszko J, Malyszko JS, Gajewska H, et al. Serum hepcidin—a protective and inverse biomarker of CI-AKI in patients undergoing percutaneous coronary interventions-PCI. J Am Soc Nephrol 2013; 24:112A.

68. Bicik Z, Bahcebasi T, Kulaksizoglu S, et al. The efficacy of cystatin C assay in the prediction of glomerular filtration rate. Is it a more reliable marker for renal failure? Clin Chem Lab Med 2005;43: 855–61.

69. Soto K, Coelho S, Rodrigues B, et al. Cystatin C as a marker of acute kidney injury in the emergency department. Clin J Am Soc Nephrol 2010;5: 1745–54.

70. Westhuyzen J. Cystatin C: a promising marker and predictor of impaired renal function. Ann Clin Lab Sci 2006;36:387–94.

71. Herget-Rosenthal S, Bokenkamp A, Hofmann W. How to estimate GFR—serum creatinine, serum cystatin C or equations? Clin Biochem 2007;40: 153–61.

72. Herget-Rosenthal S, Marggraf G, Husing J, et al. Early detection of acute renal failure by serum cystatin C. Kidney Int 2004;66:1115–22.

73. Nejat M, Pickering JW, Walker RJ, et al. Rapid detection of acute kidney injury by plasma cystatin C in the intensive care unit. Nephrol Dial Transplant 2010;25:3283–9.

74. Hoek FJ, Kemperman FA, Krediet RT. A comparison between cystatin C, plasma creatinine and the Cockcroft and Gault formula for the estimation of glomerular filtration rate. Nephrol Dial Transplant 2003;18:2024–31.

75. Knight EL, Verhave JC, Spiegelman D, et al. Factors influencing serum cystatin C levels other than renal function and the impact on renal function measurement. Kidney Int 2004;65:1416–21.

76. Liebetrau C, Gaede L, Doerr O, et al. Neutrophil gelatinase-associated lipocalin (NGAL) for the early detection of contrast-induced nephropathy after percutaneous coronary intervention. Scand J Clin Lab Invest 2014;74:81–8.

77. Alharazy SM, Kong N, Saidin R, et al. Serum neutrophil gelatinase-associated lipocalin and cystatin C are early biomarkers of contrast-induced nephropathy after coronary angiography in patients with chronic kidney disease. Angiology 2014;65:436–42.

78. Bachorzewska-Gajewska H, Malyszko J, Sitniewska E, et al. Neutrophil-gelatinase-associated lipocalin and renal function after percutaneous coronary interventions. Am J Nephrol 2006; 26:287–92.

79. Malyszko J, Bachorzewska-Gajewska H, Poniatowski B, et al. Urinary and serum biomarkers after cardiac catheterization in diabetic patients with stable angina and without severe chronic kidney disease. Ren Fail 2009;31:910–9.

80. Shaker OG, El-Shehaby A, El-Khatib M. Early diagnostic markers for contrast nephropathy in patients undergoing coronary angiography. Angiology 2010;61:731–6.

81. Bachorzewska-Gajewska H, Poniatowski B, Dobrzycki S. NGAL (neutrophil gelatinase associated lipocalin) and L-FABP after percutaneous coronary interventions due to unstable angina in patients with normal serum creatinine. Adv Med Sci 2009;54:221–4.

82. Hirsch R, Dent C, Pfriem H, et al. NGAL is an early predictive biomarker of contrast-induced nephropathy in children. Pediatr Nephrol 2007;22: 2089–95.

83. Ling W, Zhaohui N, Ben H, et al. Urinary IL-18 and NGAL as early predictive biomarkers in contrast-induced nephropathy after coronary angiography. Nephron Clin Pract 2008;108(3):c176–81.

84. Lacquaniti A, Buemi F, Lupica R, et al. Can neutrophil gelatinase-associated lipocalin help depict early contrast material-induced nephropathy? Radiology 2013;267:86–93.

85. Tasanarong A, Hutayanon P, Piyayotai D. Urinary neutrophil gelatinase-associated lipocalin predicts the severity of contrast-induced acute kidney injury in chronic kidney disease patients undergoing elective coronary procedures. BMC Nephrol 2013;14:270.

86. Rickli H, Benou K, Ammann P, et al. Time course of serial cystatin C levels in comparison with serum creatinine after application of radiocontrast media. Clin Nephrol 2004;61:98–102.

87. Bachorzewska-Gajewska H, Malyszko J, Sitniewska E, et al. NGAL (neutrophil gelatinase-associated lipocalin) and cystatin C: are they good predictors of contrast nephropathy after percutaneous coronary interventions in patients with stable angina and normal serum creatinine? Int J Cardiol 2008;127:290–1.

88. Briguori C, Visconti G, Rivera NV, et al. Cystatin C and contrast-induced acute kidney injury. Circulation 2010;121:2117–22.

89. Bulent Gul CB, Gullulu M, Oral B, et al. Urinary IL-18: a marker of contrast-induced nephropathy following percutaneous coronary intervention? Clin Biochem 2008;41:544–7.

90. Kato K, Sato N, Yamamoto T, et al. Valuable markers for contrast-induced nephropathy in patients undergoing cardiac catheterization. Circ J 2008;72:1499–505.

91. Nakamura T, Sugaya T, Node K, et al. Urinary excretion of liver-type fatty acid-binding protein in contrast medium-induced nephropathy. Am J Kidney Dis 2006;47:439–44.

92. Manabe K, Kamihata H, Motohiro M, et al. Urinary liver-type fatty acid-binding protein level as a predictive biomarker of contrast-induced acute kidney injury. Eur J Clin Invest 2012;42:557–63.

93. Duranay M, Segall L, Sen N, et al. Bone morphogenic protein-7 serum level decreases significantly in patients with contrast-induced nephropathy. Int Urol Nephrol 2011;43:807–12.

94. Vanmassenhove J, Vanholder R, Nagler E, et al. Urinary and serum biomarkers for the diagnosis of acute kidney injury: an in-depth review of the literature. Nephrol Dial Transplant 2013;28:254–73.

95. Stillman IE, Lima EQ, Burdmann EA. Renal biopsies in acute kidney injury: who are we missing? Clin J Am Soc Nephrol 2008;3:647–8.

Intravenous and Oral Hydration
Approaches, Principles, and Differing Regimens

Igor Rojkovskiy, MD, Richard Solomon, MD*

KEYWORDS

- Contrast-induced nephropathy • Saline • Forced diuresis • Furosemide • Bicarbonate

KEY POINTS

- Correct volume depletion before administration of contrast in all patients.
- Encourage diuresis with oral ingestion of water before and after contrast administration in all patients.
- In high-risk patients, intravenous sodium chloride is recommended, starting 2 to 4 hours before contrast administration and continuing for at least 6 hours after contrast administration.
- In high-risk patients, the use of sodium bicarbonate may be justified when time does not permit administration of sodium chloride.

INTRODUCTION

The administration of oral and intravenous (IV) fluids before, during, and after exposure to iodinated contrast media (CM) for the prevention of acute kidney injury (contrast-induced nephropathy [CIN]) has a long history in clinical medicine. It is now part of the guidelines of the American Heart Association, American College of Cardiology, Society for Cardiovascular Angiography and Intervention,[1] and European Society of Urogenital Radiology.[2] However, these recommendations do not specify the amount, type, or route of administration of fluid. Recent surveys suggest that only about two-thirds of high-risk patients receive hydration per the guidelines.[3] In this review, the rationale for the administration of fluid is discussed and then the results of clinical trials are considered, comparing different amounts, types, and routes of fluid administration.

TERMS

Before discussing the details of fluid administration, common terms used in this review require comment. The term volume, as used in volume expansion, refers to isotonic fluid. Several isotonic fluids are approved for use in clinical medicine: normal or 0.9% sodium chloride, D5W (5% dextrose in water), Ringer lactate, and so forth. However, only fluids containing sodium as the major solute are isotonic in the body. Furthermore, isotonic sodium-containing solutions have a volume of distribution in the extracellular space, approximately 20% of total body weight. On the other hand, the glucose in D5W is metabolized, leaving only water behind. The volume of distribution for water is 60% of total body weight. Three times more water is required compared with isotonic sodium solutions to produce the same expansion of the extracellular space. Therefore,

The authors have nothing to disclose.

Division of Nephrology and Hypertension, Fletcher Allen Health Care, University of Vermont College of Medicine, UHC 2309, 1 South Prospect Street, Burlington, VT 05401, USA

* Corresponding author.

E-mail address: richard.solomon@vtmednet.org

Intervent Cardiol Clin 3 (2014) 393–404

http://dx.doi.org/10.1016/j.iccl.2014.03.009

2211-7458/14/$ – see front matter © 2014 Elsevier Inc. All rights reserved.

in practical as well as clinical terms, volume (whether depletion or expansion) refers to isotonic sodium-containing fluid.

The term hydration is frequently used in the literature to mean volume. It more correctly refers to water surfeits and deficits, as in overhydration or dehydration, respectively. As noted earlier, the volume of distribution of water is 3 times that of sodium. Therefore, more water needs to be administered to provide comparable expansion of the extracellular (including the intravascular) space.

PATHOPHYSIOLOGY OF CM NEPHROTOXICITY

CM causes nephrotoxicity through direct effects on renal tubule cells.[4–6] The higher the urinary concentration of CM and the longer the CM remains in contact with tubule cells, the greater the likelihood of injury. CM is fully filtered at the glomerulus, and the initial urinary concentration is identical to that of plasma. However, as CM moves along the nephron, solute and water are reabsorbed without CM, resulting in an increase in the concentration of CM within the tubule lumen. The concentration can easily increase to 100-fold the plasma concentration. The degree to which CM are concentrated in the tubule lumen depends on the amount of solute and water reabsorbed.

CM also can upset the balance between O_2 use and O_2 delivery within the kidney. The medulla receives only ~5% of the total blood flow to the kidney[7] but is the location of the thick ascending limb of Henle (TAH) and S3 segments of the proximal tubule, where active transport of sodium requires high amounts of adenosine triphosphate and oxygen. Because of the unique vascular arrangement of the vasa recta that supply blood to this area, an oxygen diffusion gradient exists between the closely approximated descending (O_2 rich) and ascending (O_2 poor) vasa recta. This situation results in diffusion of O_2 from the descending to the ascending vasa recta, which further reduces the absolute amount of O_2 delivered into the medulla. The net result is that under resting conditions, O_2 tissue levels in the cortex are ~40 mm Hg, whereas in the medulla, levels ~15 to 20 mm Hg are found. An increase in solute delivery to the TAH (as might occur with osmotic diuresis) or inhibition of active transport by the TAH (as might occur with the use of a loop diuretic) can dramatically alter O_2 consumption.[8]

CM, with osmolalities higher than plasma, result in the delivery of more solute to the loop of Henle and distal tubule sites (osmotic diuresis). This situation could increase O_2 consumption in those nephron segments. The delivery of more solute to the macula densa would activate tubuloglomerular feedback mechanisms, resulting in a decrease in blood flow to the vasa recta (mediated by increased adenosine). In addition, as the vasa recta enter the hyperosmolar environment of the medulla, water (but not CM) moves freely across the endothelium,[9] and the concentration of CM increases (up to 4-fold). At these increased concentrations, all CM cause vasoconstriction in the descending vasa recta.[10] The resultant decrease in blood flow would further upset the balance between consumption and delivery and contribute to ischemic injury.

Both direct tubule toxicity and vasoconstriction lead to the generation of reactive oxygen species and a decrease in nitric oxide availability, which amplify the damage to the tubule cell.[10]

RATIONALE FOR FLUID ADMINISTRATION

There are several mechanisms by which fluid administration could be protective of the kidney after exposure to CM. These effects depend on the amount, type, and timing of the fluid administration. These effects include:

1. Decrease in urine concentration of CM
2. Decrease in urine viscosity
3. Decrease in renal vasoconstrictive factors
4. Increase in antioxidant mechanisms
5. Decrease in O_2 consumption
6. Decrease in intra vasa recta CM concentration

Decrease in Urine CM Concentration

As noted earlier, the concentration of CM within the tubule lumen depends on the amount of solute and water removed from the urine as it moves down the nephron. In states of volume depletion, more solute and water are reabsorbed as a result of the actions of angiotensin II, aldosterone, and vasopressin. The concentration of CM increases proportionately. On the other hand, with volume expansion and suppression of angiotensin II, aldosterone, and vasopressin, less solute and water are reabsorbed, and the concentration of CM within the tubule lumen increases to a lesser extent. Thus administration of fluid, particularly when it corrects volume depletion and expands intravascular volume, can be expected to decrease the concentration of CM in the tubule lumen. Because the concentration of CM is 1 factor contributing to the direct tubule cell toxicity, a reduction in the incidence of CIN with volume expansion and high urine flow rates would be expected. Even in the euvolemic state, administration of a sodium load decreases sodium reabsorption in the proximal tubule and loop of Henle and increases urine volume.[11,12]

If the administered fluid corrects hypovolemia, an increase in glomerular filtration rate (GFR) may further increase the absolute clearance of CM and diminish the duration that the renal tubule cells are exposed to CM.

Decrease in Urine Viscosity

All CM media are more viscous than plasma, and as the CM travel down the nephron, urine viscosity increases. The relationship between the concentration of CM and viscosity is not linear but exponential,[13] (ie, viscosity increases out of proportion to the concentration). Viscosity represents the resistance of particles to movement and can increase to such extremes as to slow or even stop urine flow rate. Such increases in viscosity have been shown in animal models[14–16] and humans.[9,15,17] Studies using micropuncture techniques have shown that the pressure within the tubule lumen can increase sufficiently to oppose the hydrostatic pressures driving filtration and reduce GFR.[15,17] Thus, the administration of any fluid that results in a decrease in solute reabsorption and urine concentration of CM reduces viscosity and diminishes the pressure within the tubule lumen. This pressure also can expand the lumen of the tubule, resulting in compression of neighboring vasa recta, augmenting the vasoconstrictive effect of CM.

Decrease in Renal Vasoconstrictive Factors

During states of volume depletion, there is activation of neurohormonal systems designed to restore adequate volume. These systems include the renin-angiotensin-aldosterone system (RAAS), sympathetic nervous system (SNS), adenosine, and vasopressin (ADH). All of these systems are downregulated during the administration of isotonic fluid and volume expansion.[18–21] All systems stimulate sodium reabsorption along the nephron. Water follows the reabsorption of sodium, thus increasing the concentration of CM left behind in the tubule lumen. In addition, vasopressin increases the movement of water out of the most distal part of the tubule, further increasing the concentration of CM.

In addition to the effects of these systems on urinary concentration of CM, activation of the RAAS and SNS within the kidney contributes to the hemodynamic milieu of the kidney. As noted earlier, CM induce vasoconstriction, particularly in the descending vasa recta. Activation of neurohumoral systems that cause vasoconstriction can tip that balance in favor of overt ischemia in the vulnerable

medulla of the kidney. Animal studies have found that the descending vasa recta becomes increasingly sensitive to the vasoconstrictive effects of angiotensin II in the presence of CM.[22,23] Suppression of the RAAS and other renal vasoconstrictive influences might be expected to blunt the effects of CM on medullary hemodynamics.

Increase in Antioxidant Mechanisms

Animal experiments have shown that the state of volume depletion is associated with decreased antioxidant reserve within the kidney. Volume replacement enhances antioxidant mechanisms. Renal tissue levels of catalase and superoxide dismutase are increased in the volume-replete compared with the volume-depleted state, and markers of lipid peroxidation are suppressed after CM in saline-replete animals.[24]

Decrease in O_2 Consumption

As described earlier, the medulla of the kidney is an area of relative hypoxia, and CM may upset the balance between O_2 consumption and O_2 delivery. In normal humans, administration of a water load is associated with an increase in medullary O_2 levels as assessed by blood oxygen level–dependent (BOLD) magnetic resonance imaging (MRI).[25] This effect is blunted with aging, largely as a result of reduced prostaglandin generation.[26] The effect of a water load on improvement in medullary O_2 also parallels the urine flow rate increase. These studies suggest that prostaglandin generation, perhaps as a result of high urine flow rates, either diminishes O_2 consumption or increases O_2 delivery in the medulla. Such an improvement in tissue O_2 levels could mitigate the effects of CM. In animal models using the same BOLD MRI technique, pretreatment with indomethacin and L nitroarginine methyl ester (L-NAME) results in a marked decrease in medullary O_2 after a CM dose.[27] Inhibition of O_2 consumption with a loop diuretic (furosemide) prevents the reduction in medullary O_2. On the other hand, furosemide can also reduce medullary blood flow, probably mediated by an angiotensin II surge, which could contribute to ischemia.[8,28]

Decrease in Intravascular Contrast Concentration

CM is concentrated nearly 4-fold as the vasa recta goes from the cortex to the tip of the loop of Henle (tissue osmolality 300–1200). Any intervention that reduces the medullary hypertonicity would reduce this concentrating effect. The medullary hypertonicity is affected by salt and water diuresis,[29,30] inhibition of solute transport in the loop of Henle by drugs,[28] and comorbid conditions.

Summary

CM are nephrotoxic through effects on renal tubule cells and the vasculature. These effects are related to the concentration of CM in the tubule lumen and vasa recta, respectively. Strategies that reduce the concentration and viscosity of CM in these structures can mitigate the nephrotoxicity.

CLINICAL TRIALS

The first case of CIN was reported in a patient undergoing urography.[31] Overnight restriction of fluid was routine for such studies to enhance visualization of the collecting system and ureters. Many patients also received laxatives to facilitate the imaging, further contributing to potential volume depletion. The importance of dehydration as a risk factor for CIN was recognized in the 1980s.[32] At that time, the administration of IV fluid with either mannitol or furosemide to presumably facilitate the clearance of CM through the kidney became widespread based on several observational studies suggesting a beneficial effect.[33]

Starting in the early 1990s, prospective randomized trials of different hydration regimes were performed. Fifteen prospective randomized trials involving more than 4000 patients are reviewed in **Table 1**. Most patients underwent coronary arteriography. Only one-third of the patients had baseline chronic kidney disease (CKD), a recognized risk factor for CIN.

Fluid Versus No Fluid

Two large randomized trials included a true control group that received no fluids. Chen and colleagues[34] randomized 936 patients to no fluid versus 0.45% NaCl for 28 hours beginning 4 hours before angiography. Patients with CKD (N = 216) all received N-acetylcysteine (NAC). Only in the CKD group was an advantage of IV fluid seen with a reduction in CIN incidence (34% vs 21%). No difference in CIN incidence was seen in those with normal kidney function. Maioli and colleagues[35] compared the incidence of CIN in 300 patients with ST elevation myocardial infarction(-STEMI) undergoing primary percutaneous coronary intervention, who were randomized to no fluids or 0.9% saline, 1 mL/kg/h for 12 hours after angiography. The incidence of CIN was 27% versus 22%, P = not significant, respectively. This study suggests that the timing of the IV fluid administration may be important. A third group

that received a pre-CM bolus of sodium bicarbonate had an incidence of 12.0%. This finding could be a critical issue, because many of the hypothetical benefits of fluid administration (see earlier discussion) require hours to achieve.

Oral Versus IV

Five studies[36–40] randomized patients to oral water intake compared with IV saline. The protocols differed significantly with a prespecified amount of water (eg, 500–1000 mL before CM and 1 mL/kg/h × 12 hours or 2000 mL after CM) in 4 of 5 studies. The comparator was IV 0.9% NaCl in all studies given from 1 to 12 hours before CM and 6 to 24 hours after CM. One study included NAC in both groups. Studies with a prespecified amount of water found no difference in the incidence of CIN. The only study in which IV NaCl was more beneficial than oral water had no prespecified amount of water to be taken or documentation of the amount of water consumed. Patients who received IV fluid gained weight, whereas those randomized to water only lost weight.[39]

Dussol and colleagues[41] randomized 153 patients with CKD scheduled for coronary angiography to oral NaCl (1 g/10 kg/d × 2 days) versus IV (0.9% NaCl 15 mL/kg over 6 hours) before CM exposure (total 16 g oral vs 12.4 g IV of NaCl). There was no difference in the incidence of CIN (6.6% vs 5.2%, respectively).

An observational study by Yoshikawa and colleagues[42] involving 180 patients with normal kidney function undergoing a cardiac computed tomography (CT) angiography (CCTA) found an inverse correlation between the increase in creatinine at 24 hours and the amount of oral fluid ingested after CM. No patients met criteria for CIN. However, oral fluid intake was the only independent predictor of the change in serum creatinine.

These studies suggest that oral intake of sodium chloride or water may be equally protective as IV fluids for prevention of CIN. The issue may be less about the route of administration and more about the amount of fluid administered and the resulting urine output.

IV Fluid for Hours Versus Bolus Immediately Before CM Exposure

Taylor and colleagues[43] randomized 36 patients with CKD scheduled for coronary arteriography to IV 0.45% sodium chloride for 12 hours before and after CM exposure compared with a similar total volume of 0.45% saline given over 6 hours starting immediately before CM exposure.

Patients in the latter group were also encouraged to consume 1 L of water orally starting 10 hours before the procedure. The pattern of serum creatinine change over the ensuing 48 hours was similar in the 2 groups.

Bader and colleagues[44] randomized 39 patients with normal kidney function scheduled for CT angiography or digital subtraction angiography to IV saline for 12 hours before and after CM exposure (2000 mL total) versus 300 mL at the time of exposure. GFR measured by iohexol plasma clearance decreased in both groups at 48 hours (−18.3 mL/min vs −34.6 mL/min, respectively, $P<.05$). Patients who received the longer infusion of saline had a lower incidence of CIN (5.3% vs 20%).

Krasuski and colleagues[45] performed a similar trial of overnight versus bolus administration of 0.45% saline in 63 patients with CKD undergoing angiography. The incidence of CIN was 10.8% in the bolus group compared with 0% in the overnight group ($P = .136$).

These 3 small studies suggest that administration of fluid immediately before or at the time of CM exposure is less efficacious for prevention of CIN. The studies support the rationale for administration of fluids discussed earlier. Sufficient time to increase urine output, decrease vasoconstrictive forces, and replete extracellular volume (ECV) are required for optimal protection.

Hypotonic Versus Isotonic IV Fluid

Mueller and colleagues[46] randomized 1620 patients with normal kidney function to either 0.45% or 0.9% saline administered for 24 hours starting at 8 AM on the morning of angiography. CIN occurred in 0.7% of the 0.9% NaCl group and 2.0% of the 0.45% NaCl group ($P = .04$). Women, patients with diabetes, and those receiving more than 250 mL of contrast benefited from the isotonic fluid. However, there was no advantage in the group with mild CKD.

Marron and colleagues[47] studied 71 patients undergoing coronary angiography with isosmolar CM and compared 2000 mL of 0.9% NaCl with 0.45% NaCl given 12 hours before and 12 hours after angiography. Although no difference in the incidence of CIN was noted, there were differences in urine electrolytes and effects of ECV. Saline (0.9%) led to a 13% expansion of ECV, whereas no expansion was reported with 0.45% NaCl. On the other hand, the hypotonic fluid led to a decrease in urine osmolality. Urine output was similar in both groups.

These studies leave unresolved whether in high-risk patients (eg, those with CKD) isotonic fluid is preferable to hypotonic fluid. Although isotonic fluid expands ECV and reduces the activity of the RAAS and SNS, hypotonic fluid is more likely to increase urine output and suppress ADH.

Forced Diuresis with Furosemide or Mannitol

Four trials[41,48–50] compared IV fluid with and without a diuretic. The doses of furosemide ranged from 1.0 to 3.0 mg/kg body weight. The control group received variable IV fluids for 12 hours, 6 hours, 2 hours, or at discretion of physician before CM. In all of these trials, patients who received a diuretic had a net loss of body weight compared with those who received volume alone. Patients who received a diuretic under these conditions fared worse compared with IV fluids alone.

In a recent trial[51] involving 859 patients who all received 0.9% NaCl 1 mL/kg/h × 4 hours before and 24 hours after angiography, the use of a small dose of furosemide (20 mg) after angiography was associated with a reduction in the incidence of CIN (8.1% vs 14.1%). The benefit was similarly significant in those with CKD (n = 215; 15% vs 25%).

Interim Summary

These 15 trials support the current guidelines for prevention of CIN. IV fluids containing sodium should be administered before and after CM exposure. The data supporting isotonic versus hypotonic fluid are not conclusive for patients at high risk of CIN. Oral water may be a substitute for IV sodium when administered early. Its use can be encouraged on the assumption that it increases urine output. The use of a forced diuresis with a high dose of furosemide (≥ 1 mg/kg) is associated with a higher incidence of CIN, probably because of inadequate control of volume status.

Sodium Chloride Versus Sodium Bicarbonate

The issue of the anion accompanying sodium in trials of fluid administration for prevention of CIN has received a great deal of attention. The hypothesis behind such trials is that urinary alkalinization reduces the generation of reactive oxygen species,[52] because the Haber-Weiss reaction is inhibited under alkaline conditions.[53] More than 30 prospective randomized trials have been published or presented in abstract form. The patient populations vary from elective coronary studies to patients with STEMI or those undergoing peripheral angiography. The dose of bicarbonate and saline and the timing of administration also varied. Although it is beyond the scope of this review to discuss each of the trials, a comment about the many meta-analyses is appropriate.

Table 1
Prospective randomized trials of fluid administration to prevent CIN

Author, Year	Number	Angiography	CKD (%)	DM (%)	CM	Group A (Control)	Group B	Group C	Group D	Outcome CIN/Other	Result[a] (%)	Take Home
Fluid vs no fluid												
Chen et al,[34] 2008	936	Coronary	660 normal (A + B) 276 CKD (C + D)	Normal 8 CKD 22	IOCM	No IV fluid	0.45% NaCl 1 mL/kg/h × 12 h B and 6 h A	No IV fluid + NAC	0.45% NaCl 1 mL/kg/h × 12 h B and 6 h A + NAC	Δ creatinine >0.5 mg/dL at 48 h	A = 6.97 B = 6.67 C = 34.04 D = 21.28	IV fluid better with CKD only
Maioli et al,[35] 2011	450	Coronary	8	21	N/A	No IV fluid	0.9% NaCl 1 mL/kg/h × 12 h A	0.9% NaHCO₃ at 3 mL/kg/h × 1 h B and 1 mL/kg/h × 12 h A		Δ creatinine >0.5 mg/dL or >25% within 72 h	A = 27.3 B = 22.7 C = 12.0	IV fluid better than no fluid
Oral vs IV fluid												
Trivedi et al,[39] 2003	53	Coronary	Mixed	19	N/A	0.9% NaCl 1 mL/kg/h × 12 h B/A	No IV fluid; oral fluid intake encouraged			Δ creatinine >0.5 mg/dL at 48 h	A = 3.7 B = 34.6	Sodium is better than water
Dussol et al,[41] 2006	312	Various	100	24	LOCM	0.9% NaCl 15 mL/kg 6 h pre	1 g/10 kg of oral NaCl daily × 2 d B	0.9% NaCl 15 mL/kg × 6 h B + theophylline 5 mg/kg oral 1 h B	0.9% NaCl 15 mL/kg × 6 h B + furosemide 3 mg/kg immediately A	Δ creatinine >0.5 mg/dL at 48 h	A = 6.6 B = 5.2 C = 7.5 D = 15.2	Furosemide worse; IV and oral sodium equivalent
Cho et al,[36] 2010	91	Coronary	100	38	LOCM	500 mL water during 4 h B and 600 mL during 6 h A	0.9% NaCl 3 mL/kg/h 1 h B and 1 mL/kg/h × 6 h A	Isotonic NaHCO₃ 3 mL/kg/h × 1 h B and 1 mL/kg/h × 6 h A	500 mL water with oral NaHCO₃ during 4 h B	Δ creatinine >0.5 mg/dL or >25% within 72 h	A = 4.5 B = 22	Oral equal to IV (A vs B)

Study	N	Procedure			CM				Outcome	Results	Conclusion
Wrobel et al,[40] 2010	102	Coronary	100	100	LOCM	0.9% NaCl 1 mL/kg/h × 6 h B and 12 h	Oral water 1 mL/kg/h between 12 and 6 h B and 12 h A		Not defined	A = 5.8 B = 4.0	Oral is equivalent to IV
Lawlor et al,[38] 2007	78	Peripheral angio-graphy	100	35	N/A	Oral water (1000 mL) B + 0.9% at 1 mL/kg/h × 1–2 h B and 6 h A + NAC	0.9% NaCl 1 mL/kg/h × 12 h B/A + NAC	0.9% NaCl 1 mL/kg/h × 12 h B/A	Δ creatinine >0.5 mg/dL or 25% at 48 h	A = 7 B = 8 C = 8	Oral fluid B is equivalent to IV
Kong et al,[37] 2012	120	Coronary	Normal	25	LOCM	0.9% NaCl 1 mL/kg/h × 12 h and 24 h A	Oral water 500 mL within 2 h B and 2000 mL over 24 h A	Oral water 2000 mL over 24 h A	Δ creatinine >0.5 mg/dL or >25% within 72 h	A = 5 B = 7.5 C = 5	Oral is equivalent to IV
Fluids for hours before vs at time of CM exposure											
Taylor et al,[43] 1998	36	Coronary	100	39	LOCM	0.45% NaCl ~1 mL/kg/h × 12 h B/A	Oral water (1000 mL) × 10 h B and 0.45% NaCl at ~4 mL/ kg/h × 6 h A		Maximum Δ creatinine (mg/dL) within 48 h	A = 0.21 B = 0.12	Water B and sodium A = sodium B/A
Bader et al,[44] 2004	39	CT/DSA	Normal	15	LOCM	0.9% NaCl 1 mL/kg × 12 h B/A + oral water	0.9% NaCl 300 mL at time of contrast + oral water		Δ GFR mL/min (CM plasma clearance) or 50% decrease at 48 h	A = −18.3 mL/min and 5.3% B = −34.6 mL/min and 15%	Sodium before is better than sodium after

(continued on next page)

Table 1

Prospective randomized trials of fluid administration to prevent CIN (continued)

Author, Year	Number	Angiography	CKD (%)	DM (%)	CM	Group A (Control)	Group B	Group C	Group D	Outcome CIN/Other	Result[a] (%)	Take Home
Krasuski et al,[45] 2003	63	Coronary	100			0.45% NaCl 1 mL/kg/h × 12 h B/A	250 mL 0.9% NaCl bolus 'on call' + 0.45% NaCl 1 mL/kg/h × 12 h A			Δ creatinine >0.5 mg/dL at 48 h	A = 0 B = 10.8	Sodium before is better than sodium after
Hypotonic vs Isotonic Fluid												
Mueller et al,[46] 2002	1620	Coronary	18	13	N/A	0.9% NaCl 1 mL/kg/h from 8 AM × 24 h	0.45% NaCl 1 mL/kg/h from 8 AM × 24 h			Δ creatinine >0.5 mg/dL at 48 h	A = 0.7 B = 2.0	More sodium is better
Marron et al,[47] 2007	71	Coronary	25	20	IOCM	2000 mL 0.9% during 12 h B/A + oral water	2000 mL 0.45% during 12 h B/A + oral water			Δ creatinine >25% at 24 h	A = 13.5 B = 11.7	Similar urine output and CIN incidence
Fluids + diuretics												
Weinstein et al,[50] 1992	18	Coronary, aortic, other	100	25	N/A	Control = at physician's discretion	6 mL/kg of Hartman's × 1 h + furosemide 1.5 mg/kg 30″ B; 0.18% NaCl at 1 mL/kg/h × 6 h A			Δ creatinine (μmol/L) at 24 h	A = 2 B = 37	Furosemide worse

Solomon et al,[49] 1994	78	Coronary	100	53	32% HOCM; 32% ionic LOCM; 35% LOCM	0.45% NaCl 1 mL/kg/h × 12 h B/A	0.45% 1 mL/kg/h × 12 h B/A + furosemide 80 mg	0.45% 1 mL/kg/h × 12 B/A + mannitol 25 g	Δ creatinine >0.5 mg/dL at 48 h A = 11 B = 28 C = 40	Furosemide or mannitol worse
Majumdar et al,[48] 2009	92	Coronary	100	37	N/A	0.45% NaCl 500 mL over 2 h B and 4 h A	0.45% NaCl 500 mL over 2 h B and 4 h A + furosemide 100 mg + mannitol 25 g A		Δ creatinine >0.5 mg/dL or 25% at 48 h A = 28 B = 50	Furosemide or mannitol worse
Gu et al,[51] 2013	859	Coronary	25	21	N/A	0.9% NaCl 1 mL/kg/h × 4 h B and 24 h A	0.9% NaCl 1 mL/kg/h × 4 h B and 24 h A + furosemide 20 mg at 10 min A		Δ creatinine >0.5 mg/dL or 25% at 48 h A = 14.1 B = 8.1	Urine output increased 2 times in furosemide vs control over the initial 4 h

Abbreviations: A, after; B, before; CKD, chronic kidney disease; DM, diabetes mellitus; IOCM, isosmolar CM; LOCM, low osmolar CM; N/A, not applicable.

[a] A, B, C, D refer to the groups.

The most inclusive meta-analyses (published literature and abstracts) have generally found that sodium bicarbonate was superior to saline,[54,55] although more restrictive meta-analyses (published literature only, adequate blinding, and so forth) have not found a benefit.[56] This difference may be explained by heterogeneity in the studies themselves ($I^2 > 50\%$). Publication bias is another possible explanation, because abstracts generally failed to show a benefit.[54] One of the largest randomized trials (BOSS [Bicarbonate or Saline Study], NCT00930436) presented at the most recent Transcatheter Cardiovascular Therapeutics meeting also found no difference in the incidence of CIN in patients with CKD stage 3b, 4, and 5 undergoing coronary or peripheral angiography. In this trial, the dose of bicarbonate administered (~ 2 mEq/kg) was higher than most of the other trials. Serum bicarbonate increased significantly at 24 hours and 48 hours after CM, suggesting that the lack of benefit is not explained by an inadequate dose. A large Veterans Affairs trial (NCT01467466) involving more than 8000 patients is under way, which may provide a definitive answer to this issue. Until those data are available, the use of sodium bicarbonate can be supported by lack of safety issues, ease of use, and perhaps advantage when time allows only bolus therapy (eg, patients with STEMI).

Forced Diuresis with Volume Matching

An inverse relationship between urine output and incidence of CIN has been noted by some investigators.[42,57] In the study by Stevens and colleagues,[57] patients with an increase in urine output greater than 150 mL/h had no CIN and greater than 240 mL/h no increase in serum creatinine level. Several already cited studies attempted to reduce the incidence of CIN by forcing an increase in urine output with diuretics (eg, mannitol or furosemide).[41,48–50] These trials found a worse outcome in the diuretic group, but careful attention to volume was lacking and most patients lost weight on the day of CM exposure.

In an effort to increase urine output without producing a decrease in ECV, the RenalGuard device (PLC Medical Systems, Milford, MA, USA) was developed. This device automatically matches urine output and IV fluid intake on a drop-by-drop basis. Urine output is increased initially with a bolus of 250 mL of 0.9% NaCl followed by 0.25 mg/kg furosemide, and the device is activated. Within 45 minutes, urine output exceeds 300 mL/h and remains higher than this level for ~ 6 hours. Although furosemide was used in these trials, the dose is considerably lower than in the forced diuresis trials discussed earlier. Two prospective randomized trials with this device have both found a lower incidence of CIN compared with control patients receiving standard 0.9% NaCl[58] or isotonic $NaHCO_3$ + NAC.[59] No adverse effects on serum electrolytes have been observed. A large US registration trial is under way (NCT01456013).

SUMMARY

- There are many potential mechanisms by which administration of fluid could make the kidneys more resistant to ischemic injury from CM. Clinical trials support administration of fluid to high-risk patients as follows: start fluids hours before CM exposure when possible. Data suggest that a minimum of 2 to 4 hours is necessary for benefit.
- Oral water intake should be encouraged whenever possible both before and after CM exposure. One to 2 L of fluids is recommended.
- IV sodium chloride (isotonic and hypotonic) is beneficial versus no fluids.
- Sodium bicarbonate may provide added protection, particularly when there is not sufficient time to administer a large volume of sodium chloride.
- The use of a forced diuresis with high-dose furosemide is to be discouraged. Low-dose furosemide, particularly when combined with adequate IV fluid replacement as in the RenalGuard trials, may offer additional protection.

REFERENCES

1. Levine G, Bates ER, Blanenship JC, et al. 2011 ACCF/AHA/SCAI guideline for percutaneous coronary intervention: a report of the American College of Cardiology Foundation/American Heart Association task force on practice guidelines and the Society for Cardiovascular Angiography and Interventions. J Am Coll Cardiol 2011;58:e44–122.
2. Stacul F, van der Molen AJ, Reimer P, et al. Contrast induced nephropathy: updated ESUR Contrast Media Safety Committee guidelines. Eur Radiol 2011;21:2527–41.
3. Schilp J, de Blok C, Langelaan M, et al. Guideline adherence for identification and hydration of high-risk hospital patients for contrast-induced nephropathy. BMC Nephrol 2014;15:2. Available at: http://www.biomedcentral.com/1471-2369/15/2.
4. Andersen K, Christensen EI, Vik H. Effects of iodinated x-ray contrast media on renal epithelial cells in culture. Invest Radiol 1994;29:955–62.
5. Heinrich M, Kuhlmann MK, Grgic A, et al. Cytotoxic effects of ionic high-osmolar, nonionic monomeric,

and nonionic iso-osmolar dimeric iodinated contrast media on renal tubular cells in vitro. Radiology 2005;235:843–9.

6. Romano G, Briguori C, Quintavalle C, et al. Contrast agents and renal cell apoptosis. Eur Heart J 2008;29(20):2569–76.

7. Brezis M, Heyman SN, Dinour D, et al. Role of nitric oxide in renal medullary oxygenation. Studies in isolated and intact rat kidneys. J Clin Invest 1991; 88:390–5.

8. Brezis M, Rosen S, Silva P, et al. Transport activity modifies thick ascending limb damage in the isolated perfused kidney. Kidney Int 1984;25: 65–72.

9. Seeliger E, Flemming B, Wronski T, et al. Viscosity of contrast media perturbs renal hemodynamics. J Am Soc Nephrol 2007;18(11):2912–20.

10. Sendeski M, Patzak A, Persson PB. Constriction of the vasa recta, the vessels supplying the area at risk for acute kidney injury, by four different iodinated contrast media, evaluating ionic, nonionic, monomeric and dimeric agents. Invest Radiol 2010;45:453–7.

11. Alexander E, Doner DW, Auld RB, et al. Tubular reabsorption of sodium during acute and chronic volume expansion in man. J Clin Invest 1972;51:2370–9.

12. Granger J. Regulation of sodium excretion by renal interstitial hydrostatic pressure. Fed Proc 1986;45: 2892–6.

13. Speck U. X-ray contrast media: physico-chemical properties. In: Dawson P, Cosgrove D, Grainger RG, editors. Textbook of contrast media. Oxford (United Kingdom): Informa Health Care; 1999. p. 35–46.

14. Seeliger E, Becker K, Ladwig M, et al. Up to 50-fold increase in urine viscosity with iso-osmolar contrast media in the rat. Radiology 2010;256:406–14.

15. Ueda J, Nygren A, Hansell P, et al. Effect of intravenous contrast media on proximal and distal tubular hydrostatic pressure in the rat kidney. Acta Radiol 1993;34:83–7.

16. Ueda J, Furukawa T, Higashino K, et al. Urine viscosity after injections of iotrolan or iomeprol. Acta Radiol 1997;38:1079–82.

17. Ueda J, Nygren A, Hansell P, et al. Influence of contrast media on single nephron glomerular filtration rate in rat kidney. Acta Radiol 1992;33:596–9.

18. Franchini K, Mattson DL, Cowley AW Jr. Vasopressin modulation of medullary blood flow and pressure-natriuresis-diuresis in the decerebrated rat. Am J Physiol 1997;272:R1472–9.

19. Larson T, Hudson K, Mertz JI, et al. Renal vasoconstrictive response to contrast medium: the role of sodium balance and the renin-angiotensin system. J Lab Clin Med 1983;101:385–91.

20. Persson P, Patzak A. Renal hemodynamic alterations in contrast medium-induced nephropathy

and the benefit of hydration. Nephrol Dial Transplant 2005;20(Suppl 1):i2–5.

21. Erley C, Heyne N, Rossmeier S, et al. Adenosin and extracellular volume in radiocontrast media-induced nephropathy. Kidney Int Suppl 1998;67: S192–4.

22. Brezis M, Greenfeld A, Shina A, et al. Angiotensin II augments medullary hypoxia and predisposes to acute renal failure. Eur J Clin Invest 1990;20: 199–207.

23. Sendeski M, Patzak A, Pallone TL, et al. Iodixanol, constriction of medullary descending vasa recta, and risk for contrast medium-induced nephropathy. Radiology 2009;251:697–704.

24. Yoshioka T, Fogo A, Beckman JK. Reduced activity of antioxidant enzymes underlies contrast media-induced renal injury in volume depletion. Kidney Int 1992;41:1008–15.

25. Tumkur S, Vu AT, Pierchala L, et al. Evaluation of intra-renal oxygenation during water diuresis: a time-resolved study using bold MRI. Kidney Int 2006;70:139–43.

26. Prasad PV, Edelman RR, Epstein FH. Noninvasive evaluation of intrarenal oxygenation with bold MRI. Circulation 1996;94:3271–5.

27. Li LP, Franklin T, Du H, et al. Intrarenal oxygenation by blood oxygenation level-dependent MRI in contrast nephropathy model: effect of the viscosity and dose. J Magn Reson Imaging 2012;36(5): 1162–7.

28. Spitalewitz S, Chou SY, Faubert PF, et al. Effects of diuretics on inner medullary hemodynamics in the dog. Circ Res 1982;51:703–10.

29. Saikia T. Composition of the renal cortex and medulla of rats during water diuresis and antidiuresis. Exp Physiol 1965;50:146–57.

30. Atherton J, Thomas S. Effect of 0.9% saline infusion on urinary and renal tissue composition in the hydropaenic, normal and hydrated conscious rat. J Physiol 1970;210:45–71.

31. Bartels ED, Brun GC, Gammeltof A, et al. Acute anuria following intravenous pyelography in a patient with myelomatosis. Acta Med Scand 1954; 150:297–302.

32. Kerstein MD, Puyau FA. Value of periangiography hydration. Surgery 1984;96:919–22.

33. Anto HR, Chou SY, Porush JG, et al. Infusion, intravenous pyelography and renal function. Effect of hypertonic mannitol in patients with chronic renal insufficiency. Arch Intern Med 1981;141: 1652–6.

34. Chen S, Zhang J, Yei F, et al. Clinical outcomes of contrast-induced nephropathy in patients undergoing percutaneous coronary intervention: a prospective, multicenter, randomized study to analyze the effect of hydration and acetylcysteine. Int J Cardiol 2008;126:407–13.

35. Maioli M, Toso A, Leoncini M, et al. Effects of hydration in contrast-induced acute kidney injury after primary angioplasty: a randomized, controlled trial. Circ Cardiovasc Interv 2011;4:456–62.

36. Cho R, Javed N, Traub D, et al. Oral hydration and alkalinization is noninferior to intravenous therapy for prevention of contrast-induced nephropathy in patients with chronic kidney disease. J Interv Cardiol 2010;23:460–6.

37. Kong D, Hou YF, Ma LL, et al. Comparison of oral and intravenous hydration strategies for the prevention of contrast-induced nephropathy in patients undergoing coronary angiography or angioplasty: a randomized clinical trial. Acta Cardiol 2012;67:565–9.

38. Lawlor D, Moist DK, Derose L, et al. Prevention of contrast-induced nephropathy in vascular surgery patients. Ann Vasc Surg 2007;21:593–7.

39. Trivedi HS, Moore H, Nasr S, et al. A randomized prospective trial to assess the role of saline hydration on the development of contrast nephrotoxicity. Nephron Clin Pract 2003;93:c29–34.

40. Wrobel W, Sinkiewicz W, Gordon M, et al. Oral versus intravenous hydration and renal function in diabetic patients undergoing percutaneous coronary interventions. Kardiol Pol 2010;68:1015–20.

41. Dussol B, Morange S, Loundoun A, et al. A randomized trial of saline hydration to prevent contrast nephropathy in chronic renal failure patients. Nephrol Dial Transplant 2006;21:2120–6.

42. Yoskikawa D, Isobe S, Sato K, et al. Importance of oral fluid intake after coronary computed tomography angiography: an observational study. Eur J Radiol 2011;77:118–22.

43. Taylor AJ, Hotchkiss D, Morse RW, et al. PREPARED: Preparation for Angiography in Renal Dysfunction: a randomized trial of inpatient vs outpatient hydration protocols for cardiac catheterization in mild-to-moderate renal dysfunction. Chest 1998;114:1570–4.

44. Bader BD, Berger ED, Heede MB, et al. What is the best hydration regimen to prevent contrast media-induced nephrotoxicity? Clin Nephrol 2004;62:1–7.

45. Krasuski RA, Beard RM, Geoghagan JD, et al. Optimal timing of hydration to erase contrast-associated nephropathy: the other CAN study. J Invasive Cardiol 2003;15:699–702.

46. Mueller C, Buerkle G, Buettner H, et al. Prevention of contrast media-associated nephropathy: randomized comparison of 2 hydration regimens in 1620 patients undergoing coronary angiography. Arch Intern Med 2002;162:329–36.

47. Marron B, Ruiz E, Fernandez C, et al. Systemic and renal effects of preventing contrast nephrotoxicity with isotonic (0.9%) and hypotonic (045%) saline. Rev Esp Cardiol 2007;60:1018–25.

48. Majumdar S, Kjellstrand CM, Tymchak WJ, et al. Forced euvolemic diuresis with mannitol and furosemide for prevention of contrast-induced nephropathy in patients with CKD undergoing coronary angiography: a randomized controlled trial. Am J Kidney Dis 2009;54:602–9.

49. Solomon R, Werner C, Mann D, et al. Effects of saline, mannitol, and furosemide to prevent acute decreases in renal function induced by radiocontrast agents. N Engl J Med 1994;331:1416–20.

50. Weinstein JM, Heyman S, Brezis M. Potential deleterious effect of furosemide in radiocontrast nephropathy. Nephron 1992;62:413–5.

51. Gu G, Lu R, Cui W, et al. Low-dose furosemide administered with adequate hydration reduces contrast-induced nephropathy in patients undergoing coronary angiography. Cardiology 2013;125:69–73.

52. Barlak A, Akar H, Yenicerioglu Y, et al. Effect of sodium bicarbonate in an experimental model of radiocontrast nephropathy. Ren Fail 2010;32:992–9.

53. Wardman P, Candeias LP. Fenton chemistry; an introduction. Radiat Res 1996;145:523–31.

54. Hoste E, De Waele JJ, Gevaert SA, et al. Sodium bicarbonate for prevention of contrast-induced acute kidney injury: a systemic review and meta-analysis. Nephrol Dial Transplant 2010;25:747–58.

55. Wiedermann C, Joannidis M. Increasing evidence base for sodium bicarbonate therapy to prevent contrast media-induced acute kidney injury: little role of unpublished studies. Nephrol Dial Transplant 2010;25:650–4.

56. Brar S, Hhiremathy S, Dangas G, et al. Sodium bicarbonate for the prevention of contrast induced-acute kidney injury: a systematic review and meta-analysis. Clin J Am Soc Nephrol 2009;4:1584–92.

57. Stevens MA, McCullough PA, Tobin K, et al. A prospective randomized trial of prevention measures in patients at high risk for contrast nephropathy. J Am Coll Cardiol 1999;33:403–11.

58. Marenzi G, Ferrari C, Assanelli E, et al. Furosemide-induced diuresis with matched replacement of intravascular volume compared to standard hydration for contrast-induced nephropathy prevention: the Mythos trial [abstract]. Circulation 2009;120:S1003.

59. Briguori C, Visconti G, Focaccio A, et al. Renal insufficiency after contrast media administration trial II (remedial II): RenalGuard system in high-risk patients for contrast-induced acute kidney injury. Circulation 2011;124(11):1260–9.

Pharmacologic Prophylaxis for Contrast-Induced Acute Kidney Injury

Anna Toso, MD*, Mario Leoncini, MD, Mauro Maioli, MD,
Francesco Tropeano, MD, Francesco Bellandi, MD

KEYWORDS

- Contrast-induced nephropathy • Statins • N-acetylcysteine • Ascorbic acid

KEY POINTS

- Contrast-induced acute kidney injury (CI-AKI) is a known complication of angiographic procedures and exerts a negative prognostic impact in the short and long term.
- There is no single specific drug to treat the disease once it has developed.
- Several pharmacologic preventive strategies have been evaluated.
- Various clinical studies show a possible efficacy of certain pharmacologic agents on CI-AKI prevention in addition to the routine recommended preventive measures (ie, hydration and controlled volume of injected contrast medium).
- The evidence that CI-AKI prevention (using specific drugs) results in improved clinical outcome is limited.

INTRODUCTION

Contrast-induced acute kidney injury (CI-AKI) represents a known complication of angiographic procedures and is currently one of the most widely debated topics in cardiovascular medicine. It is associated with a significant increase in morbidity, mortality, prolonged hospital stay, and increased costs.[1] The prognostic impact of CI-AKI depends on the degree of kidney injury and the persistence of renal function deterioration over time.[2,3]

The pathophysiological mechanisms that contribute to the development of CI-AKI are multiple and not yet completely understood. However, alterations in renal hemodynamics, which lead to hypoxia of the renal medulla, and direct toxic effects of contrast media on renal tubular cells are recognized as the primary mechanisms in the pathogenesis of CI-AKI. These effects are amplified by preexisting chronic kidney disease and/or contrast-related inflammatory processes and oxidative stress causing further damage.[1]

Drugs Studied for CI-AKI Prevention

In the effort to prevent CI-AKI, several pharmacologic protocols have been tested that take advantage of their single or combined antioxidant, antiinflammatory, antiapoptotic, and renal vasoactive effects.[4] **Box 1** is a list of the principal pharmacologic agents tested for such prevention.[4–16]

To date, the results of most clinical studies and meta-analyses on the various drugs present inconclusive evidence regarding efficacy. There are issues of study bias and poor methodology in several analyses.[15] In addition, comparison of the various studies is often difficult because of the heterogeneity of designs and methods (**Box 2**). Therefore, no pharmacologic agent has been specifically recommended for prevention of CI-AKI in current guidelines.[4,16–18] The principal

Disclosures: None.
Cardiology Division, Prato Hospital, Prato, Italy
* Corresponding author. Division of Cardiology, Misericordia e Dolce Hospital, Via Cavour, 2 Prato, Italy.
E-mail address: anna.toso@libero.it

Intervent Cardiol Clin 3 (2014) 405–419
http://dx.doi.org/10.1016/j.iccl.2014.03.010

prerequisites for use of any specific pharmacologic agent in the prophylaxis of CI-AKI are listed in **Box 3**.

This article focuses on the three most studied agents: statins, N-acetylcysteine (NAC), and ascorbic acid. Particular attention is paid to evidence regarding the impact of these drugs on (1) the prevention of CI-AKI and (2) adverse clinical events (cardiovascular and renal).

The possible pathophysiological mechanisms involved in the nephroprotective effect of these specific agents are shown in **Table 1**.

This article does not include sodium bicarbonate because the method of administration comports infusion of a solution with independent

preventive effect due to intravascular volume expansion. See the article by Solomon and colleagues elsewhere in this issue for further discussion.

STATINS
Do Statins Reduce CI-AKI Occurrence?

In recent years, interest has grown in the possible beneficial effects of treatment with statins in the prevention of CI-AKI given their known multiple lipid-mediated and non–lipid-mediated (pleiotropic) effects with potential nephroprotective actions (see **Table 1**).[19]

Chronic statin treatment and CI-AKI occurrence
In 2005, Khanal and colleagues[20] first reported a retrospective study on a large cohort (28,871 subjects) showing evidence that chronic statin treatment before percutaneous coronary intervention (PCI) resulted in significantly lower incidence of CI-AKI (8.8% vs 11.9%, $P = .03$). Subsequent observational studies suggested a possible renoprotective effect of statin pretreatment (**Table 2**).[20–26] The largest meta-analysis of seven nonrandomized studies (31,959 subjects) by Pappy and colleagues[27] showed a nearly significant benefit associated with chronic statin treatment (odds ratio [OR] = 0.60, 95% CI 0.36–1.00, $P = .05$), albeit with significant heterogeneity among the studies (I^2 index 88%, $P<.0001$).

High-dose statin pretreatment and CI-AKI prevention
The first randomized controlled trials (RCTs) evaluating the possible beneficial effect of lipophilic statins (simvastatin and atorvastatin) as a preventive strategy for CI-AKI in coronary subjects produced conflicting results (**Table 3**).[28–34] Several factors might explain the discrepancies between

Table 1
Nephroprotective effects of NAC, ascorbic acid, and statins

	Vasodilator	Antioxidant	Antiinflammatory	Antiapoptotic	Antithrombotic
NAC	X	X	—	X	—
Ascorbic Acid	?	X	—	X	—
Statins	X	X	X	X	X

these early studies: small numbers of subjects, different populations (chronic kidney disease [CKD] and stable coronary artery disease [CAD]), and differences in the duration and doses of preprocedural and postprocedural statin treatment. Nevertheless, one large meta-analysis seemed to suggest that short-term high-dose treatment with lipophilic statins might provide

Table 2
Principal observational studies with statins

Study	Study Design	Subjects (N) and Clinical Setting	DM (%)	Statin Treatment (% of Treated Subjects)	CI-AKI Definition Criteria and Results of Treatment vs Control (95% CI)
Attallah et al,[21] 2004	Retrospective	1002 PCI 250 chronic statin therapy 752 statin-naïve	72	NA	NA 17.2% vs 22.3%, OR 0.72 (0.50–1.05), $P = .05$
Khanal et al,[20] 2005	Retrospective	28.871 PCI 10.831 chronic statin therapy 10.040 statin-naïve	30	NA	SCr $\geq$0.5 mg/dL or 25% at discharge 8.8% vs 11.9%, OR 0.71 (0.66–0.77), $P<.05$
Patti et al,[22] 2008	Prospective	434 PCI 260 chronic statin therapy 147 statin-naïve	37	Atorvastatin (59%) Simvastatin (30%) Pravastatin (4%) Rosuvastatin (7%)	SCr $\geq$0.5 mg/dL or 25% - 24 h 3% vs 27%, OR 0.10 (0.04–0.19), $P<.05$
Zhao et al,[23] 2008	Prospective	279 STEMI and primary PCI 56 chronic statin therapy 223 statin-naïve	NA	Atorvastatin (21%) Simvastatin (38%) Pravastatin (41%)	SCr $\geq$0.5 mg/dL or 25% 7.1% vs 20.6%, OR 0.30 (0.10–0.86), $P<.05$
Bouzas-Mosquera et al,[24] 2009	Retrospective	589 STEMI and primary PCI 106 chronic statin therapy 483 statin-naïve	72	NA	SCr $\geq$0.5 mg/dL - 72 h 15.9% vs 10.8, $P = .2$
Yoshida et al,[25] 2009	Retrospective	431 CA $\pm$ PCI 194 chronic statin therapy 237 statin-naïve	28	Pravastatin	SCr $\geq$0.5 mg or 25% - 48 h 4.1% vs 11.8%, OR 0.38 (0.17–0.83), $P<.05$
Kandula et al,[26] 2010	Retrospective	353 PCI 239 chronic statin therapy 114 statin-naïve	37.5	Atorvastatin (32.7%) Simvastatin (31%) Pravastatin (22.2%) Other (14%)	SCr $\geq$0.5 mg/dL or 25% - 48–72 h 24.7% vs 14%, OR 2.01 (1.10–3.68), $P<.05$

Abbreviations: CA, coronary angiography; DM, diabetes mellitus; NA, data not available; OR, odds ratio; SCr, serum creatinine; STEMI, ST-elevation myocardial infarction.

Table 3
Principal clinical studies with statins

Study	Subjects (N)	Procedure, Clinical Setting	DM (%)	Type, Total Dose, and Time of Statin Therapy	CI-AKI Definition Criteria and Results (Treatment vs Control)
Jo et al,[28] 2008, PROMISS	247	Elective CA ± PCI CKD (SCr ≥1.1 mL/dL or CrCl ≤60 mil/min)	25	Simvastatin 80 mg (1 d pre-A + 1 d post-A) (tot = 160 mg) vs placebo	SCr ≥0.5 mg/dL or 25% - 48 h 2.5% vs 3.4%, P = >.90
Zhou et al,[29] 2009	100	Elective CA ± PCI SCr <1.7	20	Atorvastatin 80 mg (1 d pre-A + 10 mg/d 6 d post-A) (tot = 140 mg) vs atorvastatin 10 mg/d (70 mg)	SCr ≥0.5 mg/dL or 25% - 72 h 0% vs 6%, P = .2
Xinwei et al,[30] 2009	228	PCI in ACS (UA 43%, NSTEMI 26%, STEMI 31%)	28	Simvastatin 80 mg (1 d pre-A + 20 mg/d after-A) (tot = >460 mg) vs simvastatin 20 mg/d (tot = >160 mg)	SCr ≥0.5 mg/dL or 25% - 48 h 5.3% vs 15.7%, P = .01
Lin et al,[31] 2010	92	Elective CA ± PCI SCr <1.5 µmol/L	13	Atorvastatin 40 mg vs atorvastatin 10 mg	SCr ≥0.5 mg/dL or 25% - 72 h 0% vs 4.3%, P = .4
Hua et al,[32] 2010	173	Elective CA ± PCI SCr <1.5 µmol/L or eGFR ≥60	26	Atorvastatin 80 mg vs atorvastatin 10 mg	SCr ≥0.5 mg/dL or 25% - 72 h 6.7% vs 16.5, P = .05
Toso et al,[33] 2010	304	Elective CA ± PCI CKD (CrCl ≤60 mil/min)	21	Atorvastatin 80 mg (2 d pre-A + 2 d post-A) (tot = 320 mg) vs placebo	SCr ≥0.5 mg - 120 h 9.8% vs 10.5%, P>.90 SCr ≥0.5 mg or 25% - 120 h 17.1% vs 15.1%, P = .7
Ozhan et al,[34] 2010	130	Elective CA ± PCI SCr ≤1.5 or eGFR ≥70	16	Atorvastatin 80 mg (1 d pre-A + 80 mg/d 2 d post-A) (tot = 240 mg) vs placebo	SCr ≥0.5 mg/dL or 25% - 48 h 3.3% vs 10%, P = .1
Patti et al,[36] 2011	241	PCI in ACS (UA 66%, NSTEMI 34%)	28	Atorvastatin 80 mg 12 h + 40 mg 2 h pre-A (tot = 120 mg) vs placebo	SCr ≥0.5 mg/dL or 25% - 48 h 5% vs 13.2%, P<.046
Li et al,[37] 2012	180	Primary PCI in STEMI	27	Atorvastatin 80 mg (on admission, pre-A) vs no treatment	SCr ≥0.5 mg/dL or 25% - 72 h 2.6% vs 15.7%, P = .01
Quintavalle et al,[38] 2012	410	Elective PCI eGFR ≤60 (post-hoc analysis)	41	Atorvastatin 80 mg (1 d pre-A) vs placebo	SCyC ≥10% - 24 h 4.5% vs 17.8%, P = .005 SCr ≥0.5 mg 7 dL - 48 h 3.5% vs 7.7%, P = .085
Han et al,[39] 2014	2998	Elective PA or CA ± PCI Diabetes and CKD stage 2 or 3	100	Rosuvastatin 10 mg/d (2 d pre-A + 3 d post-A) (tot = 50 mg) vs no treatment	SCr ≥0.5 mg/dL or 25% - 72 h 2.3% vs 3.9%, P = .01
Leoncini et al,[40] 2014, PRATO-ACS	504	CA ± PCI in ACS (UA 8%, NSTEMI 92%)	21	Rosuvastatin 40 mg on admission + 20 mg/d (pre-A and post-A until discharge) vs no treatment	SCr ≥0.5 mg/dL or 25% - 72 h 6.7% vs 15.1%, P = .003

Abbreviations: ACS, acute coronary syndrome; CA, coronary angiography; CKD, chronic kidney disease; CrCl, creatinine clearance; DM, diabetes mellitus; eGFR, estimated glomerular filtration rate; NSTEMI, non–ST-elevation myocardial infarction; PA, peripheral angiography; post-A, after angiography; pre-A, before angiography; SCr, serum creatinine; SCyC, serum cystatin C; STEMI, ST-elevation myocardial infarction; tot, total statin dose; UA, unstable angina.

renal protection (risk ratio 0.51, 95% CI 0.34–0.77, $P = .001$).[35] This was the first step toward the individuation of a true preventive agent.

Short-term high-dose statin pretreatment and CI-AKI prevention

The Atorvastatin for Reduction of Myocardial Damage during Angioplasty–Contrast-Induced Nephropathy (ARMYDA-CIN) trial provided the first confirmation of a protective effect of short-term statin treatment on the risk of CI-AKI (see **Table 3**).[36] In a homogeneous series of 241 statin-naïve subjects with acute coronary syndrome (ACS) and ejection fraction greater than 30% who were subjected to PCI, short-term pretreatment with high-dose atorvastatin was highly effective in reducing the incidence of CI-AKI compared with placebo (OR: 0.34; 95% CI 0.12–0.97, $P<.043$). The small size of the study population made it impossible to evaluate efficacy in subjects stratified by baseline renal function.

Subsequently, the acute nephroprotective effect of short-term high-dose statin administration was evaluated in high-risk subjects in four studies comprising more than 3000 subjects (see **Table 3**).[37–40] The Protective effect of Rosuvastatin and Antiplatelet Therapy On contrast-induced acute kidney injury and myocardial damage in patients with Acute Coronary Syndrome (PRATO-ACS) study randomized 504 statin-naïve ACS subjects scheduled for early invasive strategy (non–ST-elevation-ACS = 92%, unstable angina = 8%) to rosuvastatin or no statin treatment until discharge.[40] The study shows that (1) even a hydrophilic statin is efficacious in ACS subjects and (2) the benefits against CI-AKI were consistent when applying different CI-AKI definition criteria and in all the prespecified categories of risk, including CKD and PCI. In this study, there was no significant treatment interaction with the time lapse from statin administration (randomization) to contrast injection ($P = .73$ for interaction).

A randomized study by Li and colleagues[37] also evidenced the rapid protective effect of high-dose statin administration: 180 statin-naïve ST-elevation myocardial infarction (STEMI) subjects (without baseline impaired renal function) undergoing primary PCI were administered high-dose atorvastatin immediately before primary PCI (door-to-balloon <1.5 h) and presented a significantly lower incidence of CI-AKI than did controls (2.6% vs 15.7%, $P = .01$).

This rapid favorable effect of both hydrophilic and lipophilic statins was also evidenced in other, non-ACS, high-risk subjects. Quintavalle and colleagues[38] did a subgroup analysis of 410 stable

subjects with CKD (estimated glomerular filtration rate [eGFR] <60 mL/min/m²). They observed a lower CI-AKI incidence in subjects treated with high-dose atorvastatin (80 mg) administered the day before PCI compared with controls.

Finally, Han and colleagues[39] conducted a large multicenter randomized study on 2998 Asian subjects with type 2 diabetes mellitus and/or stage 2 to 3 CKD undergoing elective coronary or peripheral arterial angiography with or without intervention. The incidence of CI-AKI was significantly lower in subjects who received rosuvastatin compared with those who received standard care.

These five studies demonstrate that short-term high-dose statin pretreatment has an independent protective effect against CI-AKI (**Table 4**). The common denominator of these studies comprising populations in diverse clinical settings is the increased level of inflammation, amply demonstrated as one of the principal targets of statin activity.[41,42]

Can Statins Improve Prognosis?

Studies on primary and secondary prevention of CAD demonstrate that statins are efficacious and safe and do not interfere significantly with other drugs routinely administered to patients with cardiovascular disease.[41,42] Several RCTs and meta-analyses showed that short-term treatment with a statin before PCI improves short-term and long-term prognosis especially in statin-naïve subjects with non-STEMI (NSTEMI).[43–45] This clinical benefit has been mainly attributed to the drug's

Table 4
Statin pretreatment as independent protective factor against CI-AKI

Study	OR (95% CI)	P Value	Number Needed to Treat
Patti et al,[36] ARMYDA-CIN, Atorvastatin	0.34 (0.12–0.97)	.043	12.2
Li et al,[37] Atorvastatin	0.084 (0.015–0.462)	.004	7.6
Quintavalle et al,[38] Atorvastatin	0.22 (0.07–0.69)	.005	7.5
Han et al,[39] Rosuvastatin	0.58 (0.38–0.89)	.01	62.5
Leoncini et al,[40] PRATO-ACS, Rosuvastatin	0.38 (0.20–0.71)	.003	12

periprocedural myocardial protection. However, the kidneys also benefit from such statin protection, which further enhances improved prognosis, as randomized studies on statins and CI-AKI prevention suggest.[28,33,36,39,40] High-dose statin treatment is associated with fewer in-hospital dialyses (0/2140 vs 7/2147) and 30-day mortality (5/1902 vs 8/1904).[33,39,40] Episodes of acute heart failure at 30 days after contrast exposure are significantly fewer in subjects treated with rosuvastatin than in controls (2.6% vs 4.3%, $P = .02$).[39] In the PRATO-ACS study, the 30-day incidence of adverse cardiovascular and renal events (death, dialysis, myocardial infarction, stroke, and persistent renal damage) was significantly lower in the statin group (3.6% vs 7.9%, $P = .036$), which also showed a trend toward reduction in rates of death and myocardial infarction at 6-month follow-up (3.6% vs 7.2%, $P = .07$).[40]

Conclusions Regarding Statins

These studies on statins and nephroprotection lead to some interesting considerations indicating their suitability as first-line preventive therapy for CI-AKI in high-risk patients (**Box 4**).

Larger studies are needed to establish the role of statin pretreatment in elderly patients and in those with severe CKD, the two categories that are least represented in clinical studies up to now. The results of the PRATO-ACS 2 (ClinicalTrials.gov Identifier NCT01870804) currently underway should clarify if the renoprotective effects evidenced to date are due to a statin class effect or to a specific drug.

Box 4
Conclusions regarding statins and CI-AKI prevention

- Efficacious especially in high-risk categories of patients
- Beneficial protective effects are adjunctive to those obtained with both standard recommended preventive measures (intravascular volume expansion and iso-osmolar or low-osmolar contrast medium)[36–40] and antioxidant NAC[38,40]
- Renal benefits are evident after short-term and very–short-term pretreatment, such as in patients with STEMI (immediately before primary PCI)[37]
- The acute nephroprotective effect is associated with better long-term prognosis regarding renal and cardiovascular adverse events

---

NAC AND CI-AKI
Does NAC Reduce CI-AKI Occurrence?

The drug most extensively studied for CI-AKI prevention is NAC, a thiol compound traditionally used as a mucolytic agent. The rationale for the use of NAC to prevent CI-AKI relates to its capacity to scavenge destructive free oxygen radicals and stimulate the production of vasodilatory mediators, including nitric oxide (see **Table 1**).[15] The favorable risk profile, cost, and ease of administration of NAC make it an attractive prevention strategy.[46]

The first study by Tepel and colleagues[47] was conducted on 83 subjects with CKD (serum creatinine [SCr] >1.2 mg/dL) subjected to CT scanning. Administration of oral NAC (600 mg twice daily on the day before and the day of the procedure), in addition to hypotonic saline infusion, resulted in a significantly lower incidence of CI-AKI. Since this first study, many prospective randomized studies have evaluated the possible beneficial effect of NAC pretreatment, especially in high-risk subjects (CKD, ACS), using different doses of drug and different routes of administration (oral or intravenous [IV]) (**Table 5**).[15,46–89] It is not possible to draw any conclusions concerning high doses,[56,63] IV administration,[53,61–65] high-risk patients,[70,88] different hydration protocols,[73,81] more sensitive evaluation of renal damage (cystatin C-based),[80,83] and so forth. Also direct comparison between studies is difficult and several meta-analyses failed to show any significant benefit of NAC in CI-AKI prevention, even pooling studies that are homogeneous for certain key criteria (dose and route of administration).[90] Moreover, a recent meta-analysis with stratification of trials according to adequacy of methodological characteristics (allocation concealment, double blinding, and intention-to-treat analysis) showed a significant benefit of NAC in low-quality studies (relative risk 0.63, 95% CI 0.47–0.85, $I^2 = 56\%$), whereas there was no significant benefit in those high-quality studies that guaranteed methodological homogeneity (relative risk 1.05, 95% CI 0.73–1.53, $I^2 = 0\%$).[15]

Even the large, multicenter, double-blind, placebo-controlled clinical trial Acetylcysteine for Contrast Nephropathy Trial (ACT), which randomized 2308 subjects undergoing elective angiographic procedures with at least one CI-AKI risk factor (age >70, chronic renal failure with baseline creatinine >1.5 mg/dL, diabetes, heart failure, or hypotension) to receive oral NAC or placebo, did not show any significant difference in the occurrence of CI-AKI between the two groups (12.7% in NAC and 12.7% in controls, relative risk 1.00, 95% CI 0.81–1.25, $P = .97$).[15] Note that most

Table 5
Principal clinical trials with NAC

Study	Subjects (N)	Procedure (Clinical Setting)	Mean Baseline SCr	NAC Dose, Route (Duration of Therapy)	Definition of CI-AKI	CI-AKI % (Treatment vs Control)
Tepel et al,[47] 2000	83	Elective CT (CKD)	2.4	600 mg × 2, os (2 d)	SCr ≥0.5 mg/dL - 48 h	2% vs 12%, P = .01
Diaz-Sandoval et al,[48] 2002	54	CA ± PCI (CKD)	1.6	600 mg × 2, os (4 d)	SCr ≥0.5 mg/dL or ≥25% - 48 h	8% vs 45%, P = .005
Durhan et al,[49] 2002	79	CA ± PCI (CKD)	2.2	1200 mg × 2 os (4 h)	SCr ≥0.5 mg/dL - 48 h	26.3% vs 22%, P = .80
Shyu et al,[50] 2002	121	CA ± PCI (CKD)	2.8	400 mg × 2 os (2 d)	SCr ≥0.5 mg/dL - 48 h	3.3% vs 24.6%, P = .001
Allaqaband et al,[51] 2002	85	CA ± PCI (CKD)	2.1	600 mg × 2 os (2 d)	SCr ≥0.5 mg/dL - 48 h	17.7% vs 15.3%, P = .78
Briguori et al,[52] 2002	183	CA ± PCI (CKD)	1.52	600 mg × 2 os (2 d)	SCr ≥25% - 48 h	6.5% vs 11%, P = .05
Baker et al,[53] 2003	80	CA ± PCI (CKD)	1.8	150 mg/kg IV 1 h (pre-A) and 50 mg/kg IV for 4 h (post-A)	SCr ≥25% - 48/96 h	5% vs 21%, P = .045
Kay et al,[54] 2003	200	CA ± PCI (CKD)	1.4	600 mg × 2 os (2 d)	SCr ≥25% - 48 h	4% vs 12%, P = .03
MacNeill et al,[55] 2003	43	CA ± PCI (CKD)	1.9	600 mg × 2 os (2 d)	SCr ≥25% - 72 h	5% vs 32%, P = .046
Kefer et al,[56] 2003	104	Elective CA	1.1	1200 mg × 2 IV (1 d)	SCr ≥0.5 mg/dL or 25% - 24 h	3.8% vs 5.9%, P = .68
Oldemeyer et al,[57] 2003	96	CA ± PCI (CKD)	1.6	1500 mg × 2 os (2 d)	SCr ≥0.5 mg/dL or 25% - 24/48 h	8.2% vs 6.4%, P = .74
Efrati et al,[58] 2003	49	CA ± PCI (CKD)	1.5	1000 mg × 2 os (2 d)	SCr ≥25% - 24/96 h	0% vs 8%, P = .49
Boccalandro et al,[59] 2003	179	CA ± PCI (CKD)	1.9	600 mg × 2 os (2 d)	SCr ≥0.5 mg/dL - 48 h	13% vs 12%, P = .82
Ochoa et al,[60] 2004	80	CA ± PCI (CKD)	2.0	1000 mg × 2 os (1 d)	SCr ≥0.5 mg/dL or 25% - 48 h	8% vs 25%, P = .08
Webb et al,[61] 2004	487	CA ± PCI (CKD)	1.6	500 mg IV (pre-A)	↓CrCl >5 mL/min - 48 h	23.3% vs 20.7%, P = .05
Drager et al,[62] 2004	24	CA ± PCI (CKD)	1.7	600 mg × 2 os (4 d)	Mean Δ CrCl	Protective effect
Briguori et al,[63] 2004	224	CA ± PCI (CKD)	1.6	600 mg × 2 (LD) vs 1200 mg × 2 (HD) os (2 d)	SCr ≥0.5 mg/dL - 48 h	3.5% vs 11%, P = .038
Miner et al,[64] 2004	180	CA ± PCI (CKD)	1.5	2000 mg × 2 or × 3 os (1 d)	SCr ≥25% - 48/72 h	9.6% vs 22.2%, P = .04
Rashid et al,[65] 2004	94	PA (peripheral vascular disease)	1.33	500 mg × 2 IV (1 d)	SCr ≥0.5 mg/dL or 25% - 48 h	6.5% vs 6.3%, NS

(continued on next page)

Table 5
Principal clinical trials with NAC (continued)

Study	Subjects (N)	Procedure (Clinical Setting)	Mean Baseline SCr	NAC Dose, Route (Duration of Therapy)	Definition of CI-AKI	CI-AKI % (Treatment vs Control)
Goldenberg et al,[66] 2004	80	CA ± PCI (CKD)	2.0	600 mg × 3 os (2 d)	SCr ≥0.5 mg/dL - 48 h	10% vs 8%, P = .79
Fung et al,[67] 2004	91	CA ± PCI (CKD)	2.3	400 mg × 3 os (2 d)	SCr ≥25% or ↓eGFR 25% - 48 h	13.3% vs 17.4%, P = .77
Azmus et al,[68] 2005	397	CA ± PCI (CKD or DM or ≥70 y)		600 mg × 2 os (2 d)	SCr ≥0.5 mg/dL or ≥25% - 48 h	7.1% vs 8.4%, P = .62
Gomes et al,[69] 2005	156	CA ± PCI (CKD or DM)	1.3	600 mg × 2 os (2 d)	SCr ≥0.5 mg - 48 h	10.4% vs 10.1%, P = 1
Marenzi et al,[70] 2006	352	Primary PCI (STEMI)	1.03	600 mg IV + 600 mg × 2 os (2 d) (LD) vs 1200 mg IV + 1200 mg × 2 os (2 d) (HD)	SCr ≥25% - 72 h	8% (HD) vs 15% (LD) vs 33%, P = .001
Sandhu et al,[71] 2006	106	PA (peripheral vascular disease)	1.24	600 mg × 2 os (2 d)	SCr ≥0.5 mg - 48 h	5.7% vs 0, P = .24
Coyle et al,[72] 2006	137	CA ± PCI (DM)	1.14	600 mg × 2 os (2 d)	SCr ≥0.5 mg - 48 h	9.2% vs 1.4%, P = .43
Ozcan et al,[73] 2007	176 of 264[a]	CA ± PCI (CKD)	1.4	600 mg × 2 os (2 d) + saline vs saline	SCr ≥0.5 mg/dL or 25% - 48 h	12.5% vs 13.6%, P = .82
Carbonell et al,[74] 2007	216	CA ± PCI (ACS)	0.95	600 mg IV × 2 (2 d)	SCr ≥0.5 mg or 25% - 48 h	10.3% vs 10.1%, P = .5
Recio-Mayoral et al,[75] 2007	111	CA ± PCI (ACS)	1.0	2400 mg IV + 600 mg × 2 os (2 d)	SCr ≥0.5 mg/dL - 72 h	1.8% vs 21.8%, P<.001
Amini et al,[76] 2009	87	CA ± PCI (CKD or DM)	1.74	600 mg × 2 os (2 d)	SCr ≥0.5 mg/dL or 25% - 48 h	11.1% vs 14.3%, P = .65
Ferrario et al,[77] 2009	200	CA or PA ± PCI (CKD)	1.6	600 mg × 2 os (2 d)	SCr ≥0.5 mg or 25% - 72 h	8.1% vs 5.9%, P = .6

Study	N	Setting		Intervention	Endpoint	Results
Jo et al,[78] 2009	212	CA ± PCI CKD	1.3	1200 mg × 2 os (2 d) vs ascorbic acid 3 g + 2 g os (pre-A) + 2 g (post-A)	SCr ≥0.5 mg/dL or 25% - 48 h	1.2% vs 4.4%, P = .37
Sar et al,[79] 2010	45	CA ± PCI (DM)	0.82	1200 mg × 2 os (2 d)	SCr ≥20% or 0.3 mg/dL or ↓eGFR 20% - 72 h	0 vs 15%, P = .08
Kim et al,[80] 2010	166	CA	1.03	600 mg × 2 os (2 d)	Cystatin C ≥25% - 72 h	5% vs 15.1%, P<.05
Thiele et al,[81] 2010	251	Primary PCI (STEMI)	0.9	6 g IV (24 h infusion)	SCr >25% - 72 h	14% vs 20%, P = .28
Sadat et al,[82] 2011	40	PA (peripheral vascular disease)	NA	600 mg × 2 os (2 d)	Mean Δ SCr - 72 h	5% vs 15%, P = .33
Berwanger et al,[15] 2011	2308	CA or PA ± PCI (at least 1 CI-AKI risk factor)	1.2	1200 mg × 2 os (2 d)	SCr ≥25% - 48/96 h	12.7% vs 12.7%, P = .97
Droppa et al,[83] 2011	251	Primary PCI (STEMI)	0.9	1200 mg × 2 os (2 d)	Cystatin C ≥25% - 72 h	74.6% vs 70.4%, P = .46
Tanaka et al,[84] 2011	76	Primary PCI (STEMI)	0.84	705 mg × 2 os (2 d)	SCr ≥25% - 72 h	5.3% vs 13.2%, P = .21
Awal et al,[85] 2011	100	CA ± PCI (CKD)	1.5	600 mg × 2 os (2 d)	SCr ≥0.5 mg/dL or 25% - 48 h	0 vs 12%, P = .012
Koc et al,[86] 2012	220	CA ± PCI (CKD)	1.3	1200 mg × 2 IV + HD hydration vs HD hydration vs LD hydration	SCr ≥0.5 mg/dL or 25% - 48 h	2.5% vs 16.3% (HD) vs 10% (LD), P = .012
Jaffery et al,[87] 2012	398	CA ± PCI (ACS)	1.08	6 g IV (24 h infusion)	SCr ≥25% - 72 h	16% vs 13%, P = .40
Traub et al,[88] 2013	357	Emergency CT		3 g IV (bolus) + 4.8 g IV (24 h infusion)	SCr ≥0.5 mg/dL or 25% - 48/72 h	7.6% vs 7.0%, P = NS
Brueck et al,[46] 2013	397 of 520[a]	CA ± PCI (CKD)	1.5	600 mg × 2 IV (24 h and 1 h pre-A) vs placebo	SCr ≥0.5 mg - 72 h	27.6% vs 32.1%, P = .20
Albabtain et al,[89] 2013	128 of 243[a]	CA ± PCI (CKD or DM)	1.29	600 mg × 2 os (2 d) vs placebo	SCr ≥25% or 0.5 mg -96/120 h	8.5% vs 7.7%, P = .684

Abbreviations: CA, coronary angiography; CrCl, creatinine clearance; DM, diabetes mellitus; HD, high-dose; LD, low-dose; NA, data not available; os, orally; PA, peripheral angiography; post-A, after angiography; pre-A, before angiography.
[a] Subjects included in a study with multiple arms.

Table 6
Guideline recommendations for N-acetylcysteine

Recommendation	Class of Recommendation	LOE	Guideline (Reference)
Use of NAC with isotonic solution in subjects at increased risk	2	D	KDIGO for AKI[16]
Pharmacologic prophylaxis (NAC and other drugs)	IIb	A	ESUR for CI-AKI[4]
Administration of NAC	III	A	ACC, AHA, SCAI for PCI[17]
Administration of NAC	IIb	A	ESC for PCI[18]

Abbreviations: ACC, American College of Cardiology; AHA, American Heart Association; ESC, European Society of Cardiology; ESUR, European Society of Urogenital Radiology; KDIGO, Kidney Disease Improving Global Outcomes; LOE, level of evidence; SCAI, Society for Cardiovascular Angiography and Interventions.

enrolled subjects (98%) also received periprocedural hydration with 0.9% saline solution.

The results of this study have been considered in most of the current guidelines that, albeit with discrepancies, do not support the use of this drug as preventive treatment of CI-AKI (**Table 6**).[4,16–18] There have been various criticisms of this ACT study: the low percentage (15.7%) of subjects with severe CKD, the inadequate definition of CI-AKI, the baseline creatinine value measured up to 90 days before angiography, and the administration of high-osmolarity contrast medium in 22% of subjects.[91] Nevertheless, the large size of the study and the absence of any signal of benefit with NAC has resulted in a marked decline in use of NAC for prevention of CI-AKI.

Notwithstanding the various limitations, the debate about the efficacy of NAC in CI-AKI prevention continues and there is strong interest in the forthcoming results of the Prevention of Serious Adverse Events following Angiography (PRESERVE) trial (**Box 5**).[91]

Does NAC Improve Prognosis?

Few studies have evaluated the impact of NAC as pharmacologic strategy against CI-AKI with clinically relevant endpoints.[15,46,78,81,84,87] Overall, there were relatively small numbers of adverse events (mortality and need for dialysis) at 30 days.

In the ACT trial, the incidence of the composite outcome of 30-day death or need for dialysis (secondary endpoints) was 2.2% in the NAC group and 2.3% in controls (hazard ratio 0.97, 95% CI 0.56–1.69, $P = .92$). Cardiovascular death at 30 days was also similar in the two groups. These results were consistent in all the prespecified subgroups evaluated, including subjects with renal failure (baseline creatinine >1.5 mg/dL), diabetes, and those who received higher volumes of contrast medium.[15]

The last meta-analysis comprising 27 RCTs that evaluated clinical endpoints (including the ACT

trial) showed that NAC does not exert any significant benefit in terms of renal function, need for dialysis, and all-cause mortality.[90]

ASCORBIC ACID AND CI-AKI
Does Ascorbic Acid Reduce CI-AKI Occurrence?

Ascorbic acid has been used largely as a dietary supplement. Today there is strong evidence that it acts as a potent water-soluble antioxidant that scavenges reactive oxygen compounds.[92] Preclinical studies suggest that ascorbic acid may also increase nitric oxide availability and alkalize the urine.[93] These facts explain why this substance has been used as CI-AKI preventive strategy. Moreover, commonly used dosages present a very low-risk profile.[46]

The nephroprotective effect of ascorbic acid was tested in a few RCTs with conflicting results (**Table 7**).[46,78,89,94–96] The six principal RCTs are

---

Box 5
PRESERVE Trial (currently underway)

- Multicenter, randomized, double-blind with a 2 × 2 factorial design comparing IV isotonic saline with IV isotonic sodium bicarbonate and oral NAC with oral placebo

- Elective or urgent coronary or noncoronary angiography

- Enrollment: 8680 subjects with baseline eGFR <60 mL/min/1.73 m^2 plus diabetes, or baseline eGFR <45 mL/min/1.73 m^2 independent of diabetic status

- Primary hypotheses: (1) bicarbonate more effective than saline and (2) NAC more effective than placebo

- Primary endpoint: 90-day clinical outcome (composite outcome of death, need for dialysis, or persistent decline in renal function)

- Secondary endpoint: development of CI-AKI

Table 7
Principal clinical trials with ascorbic acid

Study	Subjects (N)	Ascorbic Acid Dose	Definition of CI-AKI	CI-AKI % (Treatment vs Control)
Spargias et al,[94] 2004	231	3 g os (2 h pre-A) + 2 g × 2 (post-A) vs placebo	SCr ≥25% or 0.5 mg/dL - 48/120 h	9.3% vs 20%, $P = .02$
Boscheri et al,[95] 2007	143	1 g os (20 min pre-A) vs placebo	SCr ≥25% - 144 h	6.7% vs 4.3%, $P = $ NS
Jo et al,[78] 2009, NASPI	212	3 g + 2 g os (pre-A) + 2 g (post-A) vs NAC 1200 mg × 2 os (2 d)	SCr ≥25% or 0.5 mg/dL - 48 h	1.2% vs 4.4%, $P = .37$
Zhou & Chen,[96] 2012	156	3 g IV (pre-A) + 1 g × 2 after-A (2 d) vs placebo	SCr ≥25% or 0.5 mg/dL - 48 h	5.4% vs 6.3%, $P = .69$
Brueck et al,[46] 2013	300 of 520[a]	500 mg IV (24 h and 1 h pre-A) vs placebo	SCr ≥0.5 mg/dL - 72 h	24.5% vs 32.1%, $P = .11$
Albabtain et al,[89] 2013	123 of 243[a]	3 g os (2 h pre-A) + 2 g × 2 (post-A) vs placebo	SCr ≥25% or 0.5 mg/dL - 96/120 h	3.6% vs 7.7%, $P = .684$

Abbreviations: post-A, after angiography; pre-A, before angiography.
[a] Subjects included in a study with multiple arms.

based mostly on small cohorts and are difficult to compare given the differences in dosages, methodology, and in particular control treatments. Note, however, that in the recent meta-analysis by Sadat and colleagues[92] pooling nine RCTs (three abstracts and six RCTs, 1536 subjects), ascorbic acid administered preangiographic and postangiographic procedure was more efficacious than control treatments in limiting CI-AKI occurrence in subjects with preexisting renal impairment.

Does Ascorbic Acid Improve Prognosis?

Only few studies on ascorbic acid and nephroprotection have also evaluated adverse clinical outcome and time of hospitalization as secondary endpoints. Three of the nine studies included in Sadat's meta-analysis evaluated the in-hospital clinical outcome and found no significant differences between treatment arms and controls.[46,78,96] Only one study evaluated the cumulative composite outcome at 6 months (death, myocardial infarction, revascularization, stroke, and dialysis) and, again, there were no significant differences between the two randomized groups, ascorbic acid and NAC (6.9% vs 5.2%, respectively; $P = .748$).[78]

SUMMARY

Although NAC and ascorbic acid present favorable safety profile and contained costs, current data indicate that only statins should be considered

the best pharmacologic strategy for CI-AKI prevention.

REFERENCES

1. McCullough PA. Contrast-induced acute kidney injury. J Am Coll Cardiol 2008;51:1419–28.
2. James MT, Ghali WA, Knudtson ML, et al, Alberta Provincial Project for Outcome Assessment in Coronary Heart Disease (APPROACH) Investigators. Associations between acute kidney injury and cardiovascular and renal outcomes after coronary angiography. Circulation 2011;123:409–16.
3. Maioli M, Toso A, Leoncini M, et al. Persistent renal damage after contrast-induced acute kidney injury: incidence, evolution, risk factors, and prognosis. Circulation 2012;125:3099–107.
4. Stacul F, van der Molen AJ, Reimer P, et al, Contrast Media Safety Committee of European Society of Urogenital Radiology (ESUR). Contrast induced nephropathy: updated ESUR Contrast Media Safety Committee guidelines. Eur Radiol 2011;21:2527–41.
5. Stone G, McCollough P, Tumlin J, et al. Fenoldopam mesylate for the prevention of contrast-induced nephropathy: a randomized controlled trial. JAMA 2003;290:2284–91.
6. Gare M, Haviv YS, Ben-Yehuda A, et al. The renal effect of low-dose dopamine in high-risk patients undergoing coronary angiography. J Am Coll Cardiol 1999;34:1682–8.
7. Wang YXJ, Jia YF, Chen KM, et al. Radiographic contrast media induced nephropathy: experimental

observations and the protective effect of calcium channel blockers. Br J Radiol 2001;74:1103–8.

8. Morikawa S, Sone T, Tsuboi H, et al. Renal protective effects and the prevention of contrast-induced nephropathy by atrial natriuretic peptide. J Am Coll Cardiol 2009;53:1040–6.

9. Solomon R, Wermer C, Mann D, et al. Effect of saline, mannitol, and furosemide on acute decreases in renal function induced by radiocontrast agents. N Engl J Med 1994;331:1416–20.

10. Wang M, Holcslaw T, Bashore TM, et al. Exacerbation of radiocontrast nephrotoxicity by endothelin antagonism. Kidney Int 2000;57:1875–80.

11. Spargias K, Adreanides E, Demerouti E, et al. Iloprost prevents contrast-induced nephropathy in patients with renal dysfunction undergoing coronary angiography or intervention. Circulation 2009;120:1793–9.

12. Ribichini F, Gambaro A, Pighi M, et al. Effects of prednisone on biomarkers of tubular damage induced by radiocontrast in interventional cardiology. J Nephrol 2013;26:586–93.

13. Markota D, Markota I, Starcevic B, et al. Prevention of contrast-induced nephropathy with Na/K citrate. Eur Heart J 2013;34:2362–7.

14. Dai B, Liu Y, Fu L, et al. Effect of theophylline on prevention of contrast-induced acute kidney injury: a meta-analysis of randomized controlled trials. Am J Kidney Dis 2012;60:360–70.

15. Berwanger O, for the ACT Investigators. Acetylcysteine for prevention of renal outcomes in patients undergoing coronary and peripheral vascular angiography: main results from the randomized acetylcysteine for contrast-induced nephropathy trial (ACT). Circulation 2011;124:1250–9.

16. Kidney Disease: Improving Global Outcomes (KDIGO) Acute Kidney Injury Work Group. KDIGO clinical practice guideline for acute kidney injury. Kidney Int Suppl 2012;2:1–138.

17. Levine GN, Bates ER, Blankenship JC. Guideline for percutaneous coronary intervention: a report of the American College of Cardiology Foundation/American Heart Association task force on practice guidelines and the Society for Cardiovascular Angiography and Interventions 2011 ACCF/AHA/SCAI. J Am Coll Cardiol 2011;58:e44–122.

18. Task Force on Myocardial Revascularization of the European Society of Cardiology (ESC) and the European Association for Cardio-Thoracic Surgery (EACTS). Guideline on myocardial revascularization. Eur Heart J 2010;31:2501–55.

19. Davidson MH. Clinical significance of statin pleiotropic effects hypotheses versus evidence. Circulation 2005;111:2280–1.

20. Khanal S, Attallah N, Smith DE, et al. Statin therapy reduces contrast-induced nephropathy: an analysis of contemporary percutaneous interventions. Am J Med 2005;118:843–9.

21. Attallah N, Yassine L, Musial J, et al. The potential role of statins in contrast nephropathy. Clin Nephrol 2004;62:273–8.

22. Patti G, Nusca A, Chello M, et al. Usefulness of statin pretreatment to prevent contrast-induced nephropathy and to improve long-term outcome in patients undergoing percutaneous coronary intervention. Am J Cardiol 2008;101:279–85.

23. Zhao JL, Yang YJ, Zhang YH, et al. Effect of statins on contrast-induced nephropathy in patients with acute myocardial infarction treated with primary angioplasty. Int J Cardiol 2008;126:435–6.

24. Bouzas-Mosquera A, Vazquez-Rodriguez JM, Calvino-Santos R, et al. Statin therapy and contrast-induced nephropathy after primary angioplasty. Int J Cardiol 2009;134:430–1.

25. Yoshida S, Kamihata H, Nakamura S, et al. Prevention of contrast-induced nephropathy by chronic pravastatin treatment in patients with cardiovascular disease and renal insufficiency. J Cardiol 2009;54:192–8.

26. Kandula P, Shah R, Singh N, et al. Statins for prevention of contrast-induced nephropathy in patients undergoing nonemergent percutaneous coronary intervention. Nephrology (Carlton) 2010;15:165–70.

27. Pappy R, Stavrakis S, Hennebry TA, et al. Effect of statin therapy on contrast-induced nephropathy after coronary angiography: a meta-analysis. Int J Cardiol 2011;151:348–53.

28. Jo SH, Koo BK, Park JS, et al. Prevention of radiocontrast-media-induced nephropathy using short-term high-dose simvastatin in patients with renal insufficiency undergoing coronary angiography (PROMISS) trial-a randomized controlled study. Am Heart J 2008;155:499.e1–8.

29. Zhou X, Jin YZ, Wang Q, et al. Efficacy of high dose atorvastatins on preventing contrast induced nephropathy in patients underwent coronary angiography. Chin J Cardiol 2009;37:c394–8.

30. Xinwei J, Xianghua F, Jing Z, et al. Comparison of usefulness of simvastatin 20 mg versus 80 mg in preventing contrast-induced nephropathy in patients with acute coronary syndrome undergoing percutaneous coronary intervention. Am J Cardiol 2009;104:519–24.

31. Lin J, Hong LR, Qiu Y, et al. Clinical research of atorvastatin on preventing contrast-induced nephropathy in patients underwent coronary artery CTA. Clin Med Eng 2010;17:48–50 [in Chinese].

32. Hua XP, Wu RX, Yang Y, et al. Prevention of contrast-induced nephropathy using high-dose atorvastatin in patients with coronary artery disease undergoing elective percutaneous coronary intervention. Milit Med J South China 2010;24:448–51 [in Chinese].

33. Toso A, Maioli M, Leoncini M, et al. Usefulness of atorvastatin (80 mg) in prevention of contrast-induced nephropathy in patients with chronic renal disease. Am J Cardiol 2010;105:288–92.

34. Ozhan H, Erden I, Ordu S, et al. Efficacy of short-term high-dose atorvastatin for prevention of contrast-induced nephropathy in patients undergoing coronary angiography. Angiology 2010;61:711–4.

35. Zhang BC, Li WM, Xu YW. High dose statin pretreatment for the prevention of contrast-induced nephropathy: a meta-analysis. Can J Cardiol 2011;27:851–8.

36. Patti G, Ricottini E, Nusca A, et al. Short-term, high-dose Atorvastatin pretreatment to prevent contrast-induced nephropathy in patients with acute coronary syndromes undergoing percutaneous coronary intervention (from the ARMYDA-CIN [atorvastatin for reduction of myocardial damage during angioplasty—contrast-induced nephropathy] trial). Am J Cardiol 2011;108:1–7.

37. Li W, Fu X, Wang Y, et al. Beneficial effects of high-dose atorvastatin pretreatment on renal function in patients with acute ST-segment elevation myocardial infarction undergoing emergency percutaneous coronary intervention. Cardiology 2012; 122:195–202.

38. Quintavalle C, Fiore D, De Micco F, et al. Impact of a high loading dose of atorvastatin on contrast-induced acute kidney injury. Circulation 2012;126: 3008–16.

39. Han Y, Zhu G, Han L, et al. Short-term rosuvastatin therapy for prevention of contrast-induced acute kidney injury in patients with diabetes and chronic kidney disease. J Am Coll Cardiol 2014;63:62–70.

40. Leoncini M, Toso A, Maioli M, et al. Early high-dose rosuvastatin for contrast-induced nephropathy prevention in acute coronary syndrome: results from the PRATO-ACS study (protective effect of rosuvastatin and antiplatelet therapy on contrast-induced acute kidney injury and myocardial damage in patients with acute coronary syndrome). J Am Coll Cardiol 2014;63:71–9.

41. Ridker PM, Danielson E, Fonseca FAH, et al, for the JUPITER Study Group. Rosuvastatin to prevent vascular events in men and women with elevated c-reactive protein. N Engl J Med 2008; 359:2195–207.

42. Gibson M, Pride YB, Hochberg CP, et al, for the TIMI Study Group. Effect of intensive statin therapy on clinical outcomes among patients undergoing percutaneous coronary intervention for acute coronary syndrome PCI-PROVE IT: a PROVE IT–TIMI 22 (pravastatin or atorvastatin evaluation and infection therapy–thrombolysis in myocardial infarction 22) substudy. J Am Coll Cadiol 2009;54:2290–5.

43. Yun KH, Oh SK, Rhee SJ, et al. 12-month follow-up results of high dose rosuvastatin loading before percutaneous coronary intervention in patients with acute coronary syndrome. Int J Cardiol 2011; 146:68–72.

44. Patti G, Cannon CP, Murphy SA, et al. Clinical benefit of statin pretreatment in patients undergoing percutaneous coronary intervention: a collaborative patient-level meta-analysis of 13 randomized studies. Circulation 2011;123:1622–32.

45. Benjo AM, El-Hayek GE, Messerli F, et al. High dose statin loading prior to percutaneous coronary intervention decrease cardiovascular events: a meta-analysis of controlled trials. Catheter Cardiovasc Interv 2013. http://dx.doi.org/10.1002/ccd.25302.

46. Brueck M, Cengiz H, Hoeltgen R, et al. Usefulness of N-acetylcysteine or ascorbic acid versus placebo to prevent contrast-induced acute kidney injury in patients undergoing elective cardiac catheterization: a single center, prospective, double-blind, placebo-controlled trial. J Invasive Cardiol 2013;25:276–83.

47. Tepel M, van der Giet M, Schwartfeld C, et al. Prevention of radiographic-contrast-agent-induced reduction in renal function by acetylcysteine. N Engl J Med 2000;343:180–4.

48. Diaz-Sandoval LJ, Kosowsky BD, Losordo DW. Acetylcysteine to prevent angiography-related renal tissue injury (the APART trial). Am J Cardiol 2002;89:356–8.

49. Durham JD, Caputo C, Dokko J, et al. A randomized controlled trial of N-acetylcysteine to prevent contrast nephropathy in cardiac angiography. Kidney Int 2002;62:2202–7.

50. Shyu KG, Cheng JJ, Kuan P. Acetylcysteine protects against acute renal damage in patients with abnormal renal function undergoing a coronary procedure. J Am Coll Cardiol 2002;40:1383–8.

51. Allaqaband S, Tumuluri R, Malik AM, et al. Prospective randomized study of N-acetylcysteine, fenoldopam, and saline for prevention of radiocontrast-induced nephropathy. Catheter Cardiovasc Interv 2002;57:279–83.

52. Briguori C, Manganelli F, Scarpato P, et al. Acetylcysteine and contrast agent-associated nephrotoxicity. J Am Coll Cardiol 2002;40:298–303.

53. Baker CS, Wragg A, Kumar S, et al. A rapid protocol for the prevention of contrast-induced renal dysfunction: the RAPPID study. J Am Coll Cardiol 2003;41:2114–8.

54. Kay J, Chow WH, Chan TM, et al. Acetylcysteine for prevention of acute deterioration of renal function following elective coronary angiography and intervention: a randomized controlled trial. JAMA 2003;289:553–8.

55. MacNeill BD, Harding SA, Bazari H, et al. Prophylaxis of contrast-induced nephropathy in patients undergoing coronary angiography. Catheter Cardiovasc Interv 2003;60:458–61.

56. Kefer JM, Hanet CE, Boitte S, et al. Acetylcysteine, coronary procedure and prevention of contrast induced worsening of renal function: which benefit for which patient? Acta Cardiol 2003;58:555–60.

57. Oldemeyer JB, Biddle WP, Wurdeman RL, et al. Acetylcysteine in the prevention of contrast induced nephropathy after coronary angiography. Am Heart J 2003;146:E23.

58. Efrati S, Dishy V, Averbukh M, et al. The effect of N-acetylcysteine on renal function, nitric oxide, and oxidative stress after angiography. Kidney Int 2003;64:2182–7.

59. Boccalandro F, Amhad M, Smalling RW, et al. Oral acetylcysteine does not protect renal function from moderate to high doses of intravenous radiographic contrast. Catheter Cardiovasc Interv 2003;58:336–44.

60. Ochoa A, Pellizzon G, Addala S, et al. Abbreviated dosing of N-acetylcysteine prevents contrast-induced nephropathy after elective and urgent coronary angiography and intervention. J Interv Cardiol 2004;17:159–65.

61. Webb JG, Pate GE, Humphries KH, et al. A randomized controlled trial of intravenous N-acetylcysteine for the prevention of contrast-induced nephropathy after cardiac catheterization: lack of effect. Am Heart J 2004;148:422–9.

62. Drager LF, Andrade L, Barros de Toledo JF, et al. Renal effects of N-acetylcysteine in patients at risk for contrast nephropathy: decrease in oxidant stress mediated renal tubular injury. Nephrol Dial Transplant 2004;19:1803–7.

63. Briguori C, Colombo A, Violante A, et al. Standard versus double dose of N-acetylcysteine to prevent contrast agent associated nephrotoxicity. Eur Heart J 2004;25:206–11.

64. Miner SE, Dzavik V, Nguyen-Ho P, et al. N-acetylcysteine reduces contrast-associated nephropathy but not clinical events during long-term follow-up. Am Heart J 2004;148:690–5.

65. Rashid ST, Salman M, Myint F, et al. Prevention of contrast-induced nephropathy in vascular patients undergoing angiography: a randomized controlled trial of intravenous N-acetylcysteine. J Vasc Surg 2004;40:1136–41.

66. Goldenberg I, Shechter M, Matetzky S, et al. Oral acetylcysteine as an adjunct to saline hydration for the prevention of contrast-induced nephropathy following coronary angiography. A randomized controlled trial and review of the current literature. Eur Heart J 2004;25:212–8.

67. Fung JW, Szeto CC, Chan WW, et al. Effect of N-acetylcysteine for prevention of contrast nephropathy in patients with moderate to severe renal insufficiency: a randomized trial. Am J Kidney Dis 2004;43:801–8.

68. Azmus AD, Gottschall C, Manica A, et al. Effectiveness of acetylcysteine in prevention of contrast nephropathy. J Invasive Cardiol 2005;17:80–4.

69. Gomes VO, Poli de Figueredo CE, Caramori P, et al. N-acetylcysteine does not prevent contrast induced nephropathy after cardiac catheterization with an ionic low osmolality contrast medium: a multicentre clinical trial. Heart 2005;91:774–8.

70. Marenzi G, Assanelli E, Marana I, et al. N-acetylcysteine and contrast-induced nephropathy in primary angioplasty. N Engl J Med 2006;354:2773–82.

71. Sandhu C, Belli AM, Oliveira DB. The role of N-acetylcysteine in the prevention of contrast-induced nephrotoxicity. Cardiovasc Intervent Radiol 2006;29:344–7.

72. Coyle LC, Rodriguez A, Jeschke RE, et al. Acetylcysteine in diabetes (AID): a randomized study of acetylcysteine for the prevention of contrast nephropathy in diabetics. Am Heart J 2006;151:1032.e9–12.

73. Ozcan EE, Guneri S, Akdeniz B, et al. Sodium bicarbonate, N-acetylcysteine, and saline for prevention of radiocontrast-induced nephropathy. A comparison of 3 regimens for protecting contrast-induced nephropathy in patients undergoing coronary procedures. A single-center prospective controlled trial. Am Heart J 2007;154:539–44.

74. Carbonell N, Blasco M, Sanjuán R, et al. Intravenous N-acetylcysteine for preventing contrast-induced nephropathy: a randomised trial. Int J Cardiol 2007;115:57–62.

75. Recio-Mayoral A, Chaparro M, Prado B, et al. The reno-protective effect of hydration with sodium bicarbonate plus N-acetylcysteine in patients undergoing emergency percutaneous coronary intervention. The RENO study. J Am Coll Cardiol 2007;49:1283–8.

76. Amini M, Salarifar M, Amirbaigloo A, et al. N-acetylcysteine does not prevent contrast-induced nephropathy after cardiac catheterization in patients with diabetes mellitus and chronic kidney disease: a randomized clinical trial. Trials 2009;10:45.

77. Ferrario F, Barone MT, Landoni G, et al. Acetylcysteine and non-ionic isosmolar contrast-induced nephropathy—a randomized controlled study. Nephrol Dial Transplant 2009;24:3103–7.

78. Jo SH, Koo BK, Park JS, et al. N-acetylcysteine versus ascorbic acid for preventing contrast-induced nephropathy in patients with renal insufficiency undergoing coronary angiography NASPI study-a prospective randomized controlled trial. Am Heart J 2009;157:576–83.

79. Sar F, Saler T, Ecebay A, et al. The efficacy of N-acetylcysteine in preventing contrast-induced nephropathy in type 2 diabetic patients without nephropathy. J Nephrol 2010;23:478–82.

80. Kim BJ, Sung KC, Kim BS, et al. Effect of N-acetyl-cysteine on cystatin C-based renal function after elective coronary angiography (ENABLE Study): a prospective, randomized trial. Int J Cardiol 2010; 138:239–45.

81. Thiele H, Hildebrand L, Schirdewahn C, et al. Impact of high-dose N-acetylcysteine versus placebo on contrast-induced nephropathy and myocardial reperfusion injury in unselected patients with ST-segment elevation myocardial infarction undergoing primary percutaneous coronary intervention. The LIPSIA-N-ACC (prospective, single-blind, placebo-controlled, randomized leipzig immediate percutaneous coronary intervention acute myocardial infarction N-ACC) trial. J Am Coll Cardiol 2010;55:2201–9.

82. Sadat U, Walsh SR, Norden AG, et al. Does oral N-acetylcysteine reduce contrast-induced renal injury in patients with peripheral arterial disease undergoing peripheral angiography? A randomized-controlled study. Angiology 2011;62:225–30.

83. Droppa M, Desch S, Blase P, et al. Impact of N-acetylcysteine on contrast-induced nephropathy defined by cystatin C in patients with ST-elevation myocardial infarction undergoing primary angioplasty. Clin Res Cardiol 2011;100:1037–43.

84. Tanaka A, Suzuki Y, Suzuki N, et al. Does N-acetylcysteine reduce the incidence of contrast-induced nephropathy and clinical events in patients undergoing primary angioplasty for acute myocardial infarction? Intern Med 2011;50:673–7.

85. Awal A, Ahsan SA, Siddique MA, et al. Effect of hydration with or without n-acetylcysteine on contrast induced nephropathy in patients undergoing coronary angiography and percutaneous coronary intervention. Mymensingh Med J 2011; 20:264–9.

86. Koc F, Ozdemir K, Kaya MG, et al. Intravenous N-acetylcysteine plus high-dose hydration versus high-dose hydration and standard hydration for the prevention of contrast-induced nephropathy: CASIS—a multicenter prospective controlled trial. Int J Cardiol 2012;155:418–23.

87. Jaffery Z, Verma A, White CJ, et al. A randomized trial of intravenous N-acetylcysteine to prevent contrast-induced nephropathy in acute coronary syndromes. Catheter Cardiovasc Interv 2012;79: 921–6.

88. Traub SJ, Mitchell AM, Jones AE, et al. N-acetylcysteine plus intravenous fluids versus intravenous fluids alone to prevent contrast-induced nephropathy in emergency computed tomography. Ann Emerg Med 2013;62:511–20.

89. Albbatain MA, Almasood A, Alshurafah H, et al. Efficacy of ascorbic acid, N-acetylcysteine, or combination of both on top of saline hydration versus saline hydration alone on prevention of contrast-induced nephropathy: a prospective randomized study. J Interv Cardiol 2013;26:90–6.

90. Loomba RS, Shah PH, Aggarwal S, et al. Role of N-Acetylcysteine to prevent contrast-induced nephropathy: a meta-analysis. Am J Ther 2013. http://dx.doi.org/10.1097/MJT.0b013e31829dbc1c.

91. Weisbord SD, Gallagher M, Kaufman J, et al. Prevention of contrast-induced AKI: a review of published trials and the design of the prevention of serious adverse events following angiography (PRESERVE) trial. Clin J Am Soc Nephrol 2013;8: 1618–31. http://dx.doi.org/10.2215/CJN.11161012.

92. Sadat U, Usman A, Gillard JH, et al. Does ascorbic acid protect against contrast-induced acute kidney injury in patients undergoing coronary angiography. A systematic review with meta-analysis of randomized, controlled trials. J Am Coll Cardiol 2013;62:2167–75.

93. McCollough PA. Ascorbic acid for the prevention of contrast-induced acute kidney injury. J Am Coll Cardiol 2013;62:2176–8.

94. Spargias K, Alexopoulos E, Kyrzopoulos S, et al. Ascorbic acid prevents contrast-mediated nephropathy in patients with renal dysfunction undergoing coronary angiography or intervention. Circulation 2004;110:2837–42.

95. Boscheri A, Weinbrenner C, Botzek B, et al. Failure of ascorbic acid to prevent contrast-media induced nephropathy in patients with renal dysfunction. Clin Nephrol 2007;68:279–86.

96. Zhou L, Chen H. Prevention of contrast-induced nephropathy with ascorbic acid. Intern Med 2012; 51:531–5.

Device-Based Therapy in the Prevention of Contrast-Induced Nephropathy

CrossMark

Dion Stub, MBBS, PhD, Stephen J. Duffy, MBBS, PhD,
David M. Kaye, MBBS, PhD*

KEYWORDS

- Device-based therapy • Prevention • Contrast-induced nephropathy • Coronary angiography

KEY POINTS

- Comprehensive strategies are required to reduce the risk of contrast-induced nephropathy in high-risk populations and in scenarios whereby patients are undergoing coronary angiography and intervention.
- Simple medical devices have been developed to reduce radiographic contrast dose and renal exposure and to optimize hydration.
- Ongoing studies are being conducted to investigate the efficacy of these devices and to examine the practicalities of their incorporation in routine clinical practice.

INTRODUCTION

Acute kidney injury after exposure to radiographic contrast media, contrast-induced nephropathy (CIN), is a major cause of acute renal failure associated with significant morbidity and mortality.[1] The incremental presence of predisposing factors, including preexisting chronic kidney disease (CKD), contrast volume, diabetes, and advancing age, contributes significantly to the risk of CIN, which may exceed 30% in the highest-risk patients.[2] Given the frequent coexistence of some of these risk factors in patients with atherosclerosis, individuals undergoing coronary angiography or coronary intervention represent a particularly high-risk group. The development of CIN has major clinical implications, with associated higher peri-procedural mortality, longer hospitalization, and risk of permanent renal injury requiring long-term

renal replacement therapy. In this context, there has been considerable interest in the development of strategies to reduce the risk of CIN, including a range of pharmacologic[3] and device-based approaches. As reviewed elsewhere, pharmacologic approaches have yielded somewhat variable effects of the incidence of CIN, leading to increasing interest in other techniques that may be more efficacious in the prevention of CIN.

Importantly, the applicability of the various preventive interventions must also be considered in light of the specific clinical scenario. For example, the development of CIN in patients presenting with ST elevation myocardial infarction is associated with a particularly poor outcome. Given the time imperative in this patient group, only effective strategies that can be rapidly implemented and do not require a period of precontrast exposure will be practical in order to avoid any delay in the time

Disclosures: Dr Dion Stub – Supported by a Victoria Fellowship, Royal Australia and New Zealand College Physician Foundation scholarship and Cardiac Society of Australia and New Zealand Award. Prof David Kaye and Dr Duffy have research projects supported by National Health and Medical Research Council of Australia grants. The study was supported by a Centre of Research Excellence Grant from the National Health and Medical Research Council of Australia.
Cardiovascular Medicine, Baker IDI Heart and Diabetes Institute, Alfred Hospital, Commercial Road, Melbourne, Victoria 3004, Australia.
* Corresponding author. Heart Centre, Alfred Hospital, Commercial Road, Melbourne, Victoria 3004, Australia.
E-mail address: david.kaye@bakeridi.edu.au

Intervent Cardiol Clin 3 (2014) 421–428
http://dx.doi.org/10.1016/j.iccl.2014.03.013
2211-7458/14/$ – see front matter © 2014 Elsevier Inc. All rights reserved

to coronary intervention. Similarly, the use of other strategies, such as aggressive volume loading, is limited by the presence of left ventricular dysfunction or other causes of significantly elevated left ventricular end-diastolic pressure.

In this article, the authors review the various device-based approaches that have been evaluated as interventions to reduce the risk of CIN. From a conceptual standpoint, a range of device-based strategies has been developed to potentially mitigate the risk of CIN by addressing one or more of several key targets, including the minimization of contrast volume, removal of radiographic contrast to limit renal exposure, and the direct mitigation of contrast-induced renal injury (**Fig. 1, Table 1**).

Reducing Radiographic Contrast Volumes

It is well established that the volume of contrast injected during a procedure is a major risk factor for the development of CIN,[4] particularly when repeat delivery of contrast is performed early after the index procedure.[5] Within some high-risk patient populations, the risk of CIN may increase up to 40% with every additional 5 mL of contrast media used.[6] In this context, however, progress in interventional cardiology has seen the use of increasingly complex coronary interventions that require large contrast volumes; this is often coupled with the increasing prevalence of well-established risk factors for CIN in the interventional population, including preexisting CKD, aging, diabetes, heart failure, and ST elevation myocardial infarction (STEMI). Therefore, the limitation of contrast volumes should be a key objective in at-risk individuals; however, this may come at the cost of image quality. One potential source for mitigation of largely wasted contrast volume is that attributable to excess coronary ostial reflux. Although the exact amount of contrast reflux has not been precisely determined, it has been previously shown to be present in more than 60% of contrast injections.[7] Recently, a device designed to attenuate the loss of contrast caused by reflux by altering the contrast injection pressure profile (AVERT, Osprey Medical, Minneapolis, MN) was shown to reduce contrast volumes by approximately 40% without significant loss of image quality.[8] The influence of this approach on the incidence of CIN is currently being evaluated in a randomized clinical trial (AVERT Clinical Trial, NCT01976299).

The use of automated contrast injection systems has also been proposed as a means of limiting the volume of radiographic contrast[9] and possibly the incidence of CIN.[10] Recently, however, Gurm and colleagues,[11] in a large registry study, demonstrated that automated injection systems reduced contrast volumes by less than 3%, and there was no impact on the rate of CIN.

REMOVAL OF CONTRAST MEDIA

Following coronary delivery of iodinated radiographic contrast, the possibility of removing

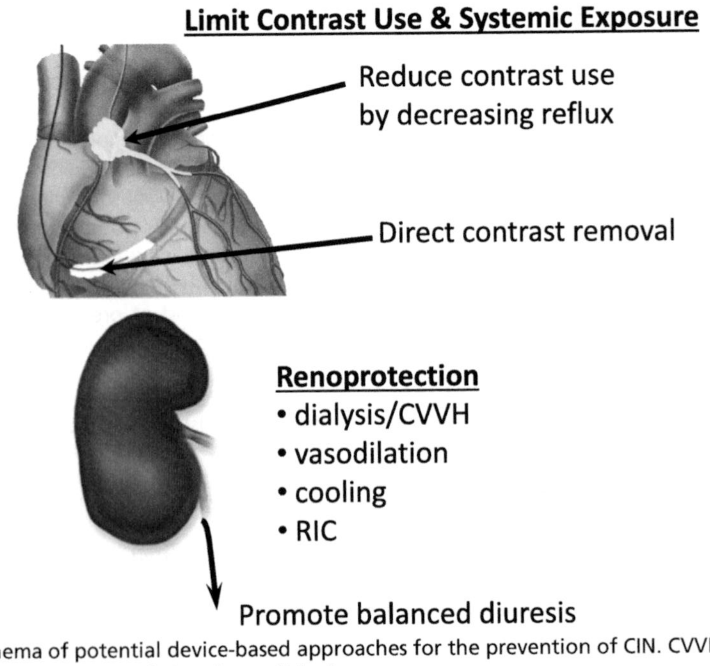

Limit Contrast Use & Systemic Exposure

Reduce contrast use by decreasing reflux

Direct contrast removal

Renoprotection
- dialysis/CVVH
- vasodilation
- cooling
- RIC

Promote balanced diuresis

Fig. 1. General schema of potential device-based approaches for the prevention of CIN. CVVH, continuous venoveno hemofiltration; RIC, remote ischemic conditioning.

Table 1
Comparative studies of device-based therapies for prevention of CIN after coronary angiography

Study	Study Design	Study Population Baseline Creatinine or eGFR	Primary End Point	Treatment Effect
Direct removal of contrast media				
Hemodialysis				
Lehnert et al,[15] 1998	Randomized	30 Patients 212 ± 14 μmol/L	Contrast removal	Average removal of 32% of contrast media; but increased rates of CIN (53% vs 40%)
Vogt et al,[16] 2001	Randomized	113 Patients 316 ± 112 μmol/L	CIN and MACE	Nonsignificant increase in event rate (24% vs 14%)
Hsieh et al,[17] 2005	Case control	40 Patients 216 ± 11 μmol/L	Short- and long-term renal function	No significant change in renal function between both groups
Continuous hemofiltration				
Marenzi et al,[20] 2003	Randomized	114 Patients 265 ± 88 μmol/L	CIN	Significant reduction in CIN with hemofiltration (5% vs 50%)
Marenzi et al,[21] 2006	Randomized	92 Patients 205 ± 50 μmol/L	CIN	Significant reduction with 2 doses of hemofiltration compared with control (3% vs 26% vs 40%)
Removal of contrast from coronary sinus				
Danenberg et al,[26] 2008	Pilot study	7 Patients 262 ± 56 μmol/L	Contrast removal	Able to perform in 4 patients, with average removal of 44% of contrast media
Duffy et al,[27] 2010	Case control	41 Patients eGFR <60 mL/min	Change in eGFR	Able to perform in 31 of 41 patients; significant improvement in change in eGFR -0.7 vs -2.5 mL/min
Automated balanced hydration system				
Briguori et al,[35] 2011	Randomized	294 Patients 99 IQR (70–216) μmol/L	CIN	Significant reduction in rate of CIN (11% vs 21%)
Marenzi et al,[34] 2012	Randomized	170 Patients 94 ± 20 μmol/L	CIN	Significant reduction in rate of CIN (5% vs 18%)
Remote ischemic conditioning				
Er et al,[49] 2012	Randomized	100 Patients 90 IQR (81–100) μmol/L	CIN	Significant reduction in rate of CIN (12% vs 40%)
Deftereos et al,[50] 2013	Randomized	225 Patients 55 IQR (50–72) μmol/L	CIN	Significant reduction in rate of CIN (12% vs 30%)
Dual intrarenal drug infusion				
Talati et al,[37] 2012	Retrospective case control	104 Patients eGFR 31 ± 12 mL/min	CIN	Significant reduction in CIN (12% vs 30%)

Abbreviations: eGFR, estimated glomerular filtration rate; IQR, inter quartile range; MACE, major adverse cardiac events.

contrast before its exposure to the kidneys has also been an appealing target. In broad terms, 2 approaches have been applied in the context of coronary imaging involving either the removal of radiographic contrast from the coronary sinus (CS) before exit from the heart to the general circulation or, alternatively, the removal of contrast from the general circulation by hemodialysis (HD) or continuous veno-veno hemofiltration.

HD and Continuous Veno-Veno Hemofiltration

Although it is well established that HD is effective in eliminating contrast agent from the blood,[12–14] this has not translated to a reduction in rates of CIN or improved clinical outcomes. In a small randomized trial of 30 patients with CKD, Lehnert and colleagues[15] found that prophylactic HD started 63 minutes after radiocontrast procedures could effectively remove contrast agent but had no significant benefit on the postprocedural change in creatinine or incidence of CIN. In a larger randomized trial of 113 patients with significant baseline CKD (creatinine >200 μm/L), Vogt and colleagues[16] found that prophylactic HD started 60 minutes after low-osmolality radiocontrast administration did not show any short-term beneficial effect compared with conservative measures, with actually a deterioration in renal function in the HD group. Furthermore, patients who received prophylactic HD were more likely to have procedure-related complications. The lack of efficacy of HD in the prevention of CIN has been further confirmed in another case control study of patients undergoing coronary angiography.[17]

In contrast to hemodialysis, continuous venoveno hemofiltration (CVVH) is a continuous form of renal-replacement therapy that constitutes an alternative strategy for extracorporeal removal of contrast following radiological procedures. Hemofiltration is associated with hemodynamic stability and may allow for significantly increased volumes of hydration, without an associated risk of fluid overload and lung congestion,[18] and can be safely performed following percutaneous coronary intervention (PCI).[19]

In an initial single-center randomized study, Marenzi and colleagues[20] studied the effects of CVVH and saline hydration initiated 4 to 8 hours before the coronary intervention and continued for 18 to 24 hours after the procedure was completed. An increase in the serum creatinine concentration of more than 25% from the baseline value after the coronary intervention occurred less frequently among the patients in the hemofiltration group than among the control patients (5% vs 50%, P<.001), although the rate of increase in creatinine in the CVVH group seemed to parallel that in the control group after the cessation of CVVH. Significant effects on the incidence of in-hospital events and cumulative 1-year survival were also observed. In a further randomized trial, the same group randomized patients to CVVH beginning before or after the coronary intervention. This study showed that although CVVH commencing before the procedure was effective, the effect of CVVH initiated after the procedure was more modest.[21] Taken together, although these results are encouraging, confirmation with larger multisite studies is required. Perhaps most importantly, the cost and resource implications of CVVH are a major limitation in the widespread adoption of such an approach, perhaps with the exception of very-highest-risk patients.

Removal of Contrast via the CS

Prevention of contrast release from the heart to the general circulation by CS blood collection is another approach that has been recently tested by several groups. The CS receives blood from most of the left ventricular myocardium and drains much of the left coronary circulation while receiving a more variable distribution from the right coronary artery. Since the inception of cardiac resynchronization therapy in particular, experience in CS cannulation has grown considerably, building on the prior experience of electrophysiologists and invasive cardiovascular physiologists.

Movahed and colleagues[22] first illustrated the concept of removing contrast via CS in an animal proof-of-concept study. In this study, the CS of 5 pigs undergoing coronary angiography were cannulated, and 50 mL of blood was collected immediately after coronary contrast injection. An average of 51% of the injected contrast was recovered by this method. In the same year, Meyer and colleagues[23] used a balloon-tipped through lumen catheter introduced via the superior vena cava in dogs. The balloon was inflated during the injections, and the venous blood from the CS was collected. An average of 70% of the injected contrast was captured by this method. Michishita and Fujii[24] incorporated a contrast-adsorbing column in conjunction with a blood-suction catheter used to retrieve the contrast material from the balloon-occluded CS in pigs undergoing coronary artery catheterization. The mean calculated iodine removal rate was 49%.

Another system involves a dual-contrast detection/aspiration system (Catharos Medical Systems, Los Gatos, CA, USA). The catheter has an expanding tip and integrated fiber optics using a light-reflection technology for endovascular contrast detection.[25] The catheter system monitors CS blood for contrast presence and provides signals for CS evacuation. A peristaltic pump that evacuates contrast-laden CS blood through the catheter's central lumen facilitates aspiration. A preclinical study reported approximately 60% retrieval of injected contrast.[25]

These preliminary preclinical models have subsequently been translated into several differing CS contrast collecting systems used in the clinical setting.[26–28] Danenberg and colleagues[26] cannulated the CS with a double-lumen, balloon-tipped catheter; however, they were unable to maintain an adequate position of the Reverse Berman catheter (Arrow International, Reading, PA, USA) in the CS reliably; but in the 3 remaining patients, 44% of the injected contrast material was retrieved.

The contrast removal system with the largest clinical experience is the CINCOR removal system (Osprey Medical, Minnetonka, MN, USA).[27] In the initial clinical report, Duffy and colleagues[27] performed a safety and efficacy study using a purpose-designed 11-F CS aspiration catheter and CS support device placed via a 14-F right internal jugular vein sheath. The CS was successfully cannulated with the aspiration catheter in 31 of 41 patients, and there were no device-related serious adverse events. In this nonrandomized study, patients with an estimated glomerular filtration rate (eGFR) of less than 60 mL/min had no change in eGFR at 72 hours after the procedure compared with a matched comparator cohort in which eGFR decreased significantly after the procedure despite similar demographics and contrast volumes. CS contrast aspiration resulted in the recapture of 32% +/− 3% of the delivered contrast, ranging from 6% to 64%. A CINCOR removal catheter for CS cannulation via the femoral vein has been developed and successfully implemented in small patient series.[29]

Together these studies demonstrate that CS collection of contrast is feasible; however, the more complete collection of injected contrast seems more challenging perhaps because of the initial loss caused by coronary reflux as described earlier.

DEVICE-MEDIATED RENAL PROTECTION
Automated Balanced Hydration

Data from the prospective randomized trial of prevention measures in patients at high risk for contrast nephropathy (PRINCE trial) highlighted that increasing urine flow rate (>150 mL/h) may potentially reduce the nephrotoxic effect of contrast media.[30] The postulated mechanism of benefit being that high urine output would lower the concentration of contrast in the kidneys, reducing transit time of contrast through the kidneys and improved flow in renal tubules. The evidence for hydration per se and the composition of the administered fluids are addressed elsewhere in this series.

The combined use of diuretics and hydration to reduce CIN have in general been associated with worse clinical outcomes,[31,32] possibly because of the difficulty in matching hydration, intravascular volume, and urine volume. In this context, an automated system consisting of a closed-loop fluid management system comprising a high-volume pump, a dual-weight measuring system, single-use intravenous set, and urine collection system that interfaces with a urinary catheter and real-time display of urine and replacement fluid volume was developed to optimize hydration and urinary flow (RenalGuard System, PLC Medical Systems, Inc, Milford, MA, USA) supported with the use of intravenous diuretics.

Two phase-3 multicenter randomized trials of the RenalGuard system have subsequently been performed.[33,34] The first was the Renal Insufficiency Trial After Contrast Media Administration Trial II.[33,35] This study randomized patients with an eGFR less than 30 mL/min/1.73 m^2 and/or a Mehran risk score greater than 11 to either sodium bicarbonate solution and n-acetylcysteine or system-guided hydration in an open-label study. The primary end point of an increase of greater than 0.3 mg/dL in serum creatinine at 48 hours was significantly reduced in the RenalGuard group (11.0% vs 20.5%, $P = .025$) supported by a significant attenuation of the postcontrast cystatin C increase. The second trial, MYTHOS, was a single-center Italian study.[34] This study randomized 174 elective patients or patients with non-STEMI, most of whom had CKD stage 3 renal disease, to matched hydration with the RenalGuard system extending from 90 minutes before to 4 hours after the procedure compared with control hydration for at least 12 hours before and 12 hours after the procedure. The primary end point of CIN, defined as a more than 25% or 0.5-mg/dL increase in serum creatinine at 72 hours, was significantly reduced in the matched hydration group compared with controls (4.6% vs 18.0%, $P = .005$), with a trend toward a reduction in a composite outcome of clinical cardiac events. Further studies of this system are presently underway (CIN-RG trial, NCT01456013).

Renal Cooling

Driven by interest in the potential protective effects of cooling on oxidative tissue injury in other organs, the possibility that systemic cooling may prevent CIN has also been addressed. The systemic hypothermia to prevent radiocontrast nephropathy (COOL RCN trial) investigated whether systemic hypothermia is effective in preventing CIN in patients with CKD. Patients at risk for CIN were randomized to standard care versus intravascular catheter-induced systemic hypothermia as a preventive strategy. The study showed that the therapy could be used safely in patients undergoing angiography; however, there was no net effect on rates of CIN.[36]

Intrarenal Drug Infusion

The influence of various pharmacologic interventions on the incidence of CIN has been discussed elsewhere. In an attempt to enhance the potential effectiveness of such strategies, the effect of direct intrarenal infusion of various agents has been investigated. Among these, a bifurcated catheter (Benephit catheter, AngioDynamics, Latham, NY, USA) has been used for dual direct renal infusion of fenoldopam, a drug that has been shown to improve renal blood flow but not CIN rates when used intravenously. A recent retrospective observational nonrandomized study showed that dual intrarenal infusion was associated with lower CIN rates than a matched control group.[37] Further studies would be required to establish the practicality and efficacy of this approach.

Remote Ischemic Conditioning

Remote ischemic conditioning (RIC) is a therapeutic strategy by which protection can be afforded to one vascular bed by ischemia to another bed in the same or different organ. Although the precise mechanism of organ protection in RIC is not entirely understood, it has been reported that brief episodes of nonlethal ischemia and reperfusion preserve adenosine triphosphate during ischemia[38]; induce production of endogenous autacoids, such as adenosine, opioids, and bradykinin that activate protein kinases so as to inhibit the opening of the mitochondrial permeability transition pore that plays a critical role in tissue necrosis[39,40]; reduce the generation of deleterious reactive oxygen species[41,42]; and attenuate inflammation.[43]

Although most RIC research has focused on myocardial protection, some studies have investigated the benefit of RIC in the reduction of acute kidney injury in the setting of cardiac and major noncardiac surgery, with varying results.[44–48] This paradigm has also led to the evaluation of RIC as a potential renoprotective strategy against CIN. A

randomized control trial performed by Er and colleagues[49] studied the effects of RIC in patients undergoing elective coronary angiogram. One hundred patients with CKD (eGFR <60 mL/min) were randomized to receive RIC (4 cycles of alternating 5-minute inflation and 5-minute deflation of a standard upper arm blood pressure cuff to 50 mm Hg +systolic blood pressure) or a sham RIC (blood pressure cuff inflated to diastolic pressure and then deflated to 10 mm Hg). The primary end point of CIN at 48 hours was significantly reduced in the RIC group compared with the control (12% vs 40%, $P = .002$), albeit perhaps with a surprisingly high incidence of CIN in controls. Using a different approach, the effects of myocardial rather than skeletal muscle ischemia was examined in another study. Following PCI, the effect of four 1-minute cycles each consisting of a 30-second stent balloon inflation to nominal pressure with 30 seconds deflation was performed in a single-blind study.[50] The primary end point of CIN at 96 hours was significantly reduced in the RIC group (12.4% vs 29.5%, $P = .002$). Larger studies with increased power are needed in these populations to confirm the effects of RIC on renal protection and its clinical sequelae.

SUMMARY

CIN is a common condition that is associated with short- and, likely, long-term adverse outcomes. Although periprocedural intravenous hydration is the simplest and most widely used technique to prevent CIN, the limited ability of this approach to mitigate CIN risk in high-risk populations, such as those patients with established advanced CKD and patients with STEMI, has provided an impetus to develop new preventive strategies. A range of potentially useful device-based approaches offers new preventive techniques. Well-designed and adequately powered randomized studies of these device-based therapies are urgently needed to determine the expanding role they will play in future clinical practice.

REFERENCES

1. McCullough PA. Contrast-induced acute kidney injury. J Am Coll Cardiol 2008;51:1419–28.
2. Mehran R, Aymong ED, Nikolsky E, et al. A simple risk score for prediction of contrast-induced nephropathy after percutaneous coronary intervention: development and initial validation. J Am Coll Cardiol 2004;44:1393–9.
3. Pannu N, Wiebe N, Tonelli M, Alberta Kidney Disease Network. Prophylaxis strategies for contrast-induced nephropathy. JAMA 2006;295:2765–79.

4. Freeman RV, O'Donnell M, Share D, et al. Nephropathy requiring dialysis after percutaneous coronary intervention and the critical role of an adjusted contrast dose. Am J Cardiol 2002;90: 1068–73.

5. Abujudeh HH, Gee MS, Kaewlai R. In emergency situations, should serum creatinine be checked in all patients before performing second contrast CT examinations within 24 hours? J Am Coll Radiol 2009;6:268–73.

6. Manske CL, Sprafka JM, Strony JT, et al. Contrast nephropathy in azotemic diabetic patients undergoing coronary angiography. Am J Med 1990;89: 615–20.

7. Franken G, Zeitler E. Experience with mechanical contrast medium injection at selective coronary angiography. Cardiovasc Radiol 1978;1:21–6.

8. Kaye D, Stub D, Mak V, et al. Reducing iodinated contrast volume by manipulating injection pressure during coronary angiography. Catheter Cardiovasc Interv 2014;83(5):741–5.

9. Chahoud G, Khoukaz S, El-Shafei A, et al. Randomized comparison of coronary angiography using 4F catheters: 4F manual versus "acisted" power injection technique. Catheter Cardiovasc Interv 2001;53:221–4.

10. Call J, Sacrinty M, Applegate R, et al. Automated contrast injection in contemporary practice during cardiac catheterization and PCI: effects on contrast-induced nephropathy. J Invasive Cardiol 2006;18:469–74.

11. Gurm HS, Smith D, Share D, et al. Impact of automated contrast injector systems on contrast use and contrast-associated complications in patients undergoing percutaneous coronary interventions. JACC Cardiovasc Interv 2013;6:399–405.

12. Matzkies FK, Reinecke H, Tombach B, et al. Influence of dialysis procedure, membrane surface and membrane material on iopromide elimination in patients with reduced kidney function. Am J Nephrol 2000;20:300–4.

13. Waaler A, Svaland M, Fauchald P, et al. Elimination of iohexol, a low osmolar nonionic contrast medium, by hemodialysis in patients with chronic renal failure. Nephron 1990;56:81–5.

14. Moon SS, Back SE, Kurkus J, et al. Hemodialysis for elimination of the nonionic contrast medium iohexol after angiography in patients with impaired renal function. Nephron 1995;70:430–7.

15. Lehnert T, Keller E, Gondolf K, et al. Effect of haemodialysis after contrast medium administration in patients with renal insufficiency. Nephrol Dial Transplant 1998;13:358–62.

16. Vogt B, Ferrari P, Schönholzer C, et al. Prophylactic hemodialysis after radiocontrast media in patients with renal insufficiency is potentially harmful. Am J Med 2001;111:692–8.

17. Hsieh YC, Ting CT, Liu TJ, et al. Short- and long-term renal outcomes of immediate prophylactic hemodialysis after cardiovascular catheterizations in patients with severe renal insufficiency. Int J Cardiol 2005;101:407–13.

18. Forni LG, Hilton PJ. Continuous hemofiltration in the treatment of acute renal failure. N Engl J Med 1997; 336:1303–9.

19. Marenzi G, Bartorelli AL, Lauri G, et al. Continuous veno-venous hemofiltration for the treatment of contrast-induced acute renal failure after percutaneous coronary interventions. Catheter Cardiovasc Interv 2003;58:59–64.

20. Marenzi G, Marana I, Lauri G, et al. The prevention of radiocontrast-agent–induced nephropathy by hemofiltration. N Engl J Med 2003;349:1333–40.

21. Marenzi G, Lauri G, Campodonico J, et al. Comparison of two hemofiltration protocols for prevention of contrast-induced nephropathy in high-risk patients. Am J Med 2006;119:155–62.

22. Movahed MR, Wong J, Molloi S. Removal of iodine contrast from coronary sinus in swine during coronary angiography. J Am Coll Cardiol 2006;47:465–7.

23. Meyer M, Dauerman HL, Bell SP, et al. Coronary venous capture of contrast during angiography. J Interv Cardiol 2006;19:401–4.

24. Michishita I, Fujii Z. A novel contrast removal system from the coronary sinus using an adsorbing column during coronary angiography in a porcine model. J Am Coll Cardiol 2006;47:1866–70.

25. Chang H, Hassan AH, Kim YL, et al. A novel technique for endovascular detection and removal of radiographic contrast during angiography. J Invasive Cardiol 2009;21:314–8.

26. Danenberg HD, Lotan C, Varshitski B, et al. Removal of contrast medium from the coronary sinus during coronary angiography: feasibility of a simple and available technique for the prevention of nephropathy. Cardiovasc Revasc Med 2008;9: 9–13.

27. Duffy SJ, Ruygrok P, Juergens CP, et al. Removal of contrast media from the coronary sinus attenuates renal injury after coronary angiography and intervention. J Am Coll Cardiol 2010;56:525–6.

28. Hassan AH, Luna J, Davidson CJ, et al. Endovascular detection and removal of radiographic contrast. Cardiovasc Revasc Med 2010;11:114–5.

29. Watson T, Burd JS, Ruygrok PN. Prevention of contrast induced nephropathy during coronary angiography with a coronary sinus contrast removal system sited from the femoral vein. Int J Cardiol 2013;165:e9–10.

30. Stevens MA, McCullough PA, Tobin KJ, et al. A prospective randomized trial of prevention measures in patients at high risk for contrast nephropathy: results of the P.R.I.N.C.E. Study. Prevention

of Radiocontrast Induced Nephropathy Clinical Evaluation. J Am Coll Cardiol 1999;33:403–11.

31. Solomon R, Werner C, Mann D, et al. Effects of saline, mannitol, and furosemide to prevent acute decreases in renal function induced by radiocontrast agents. N Engl J Med 1994;331:1416–20.

32. Dussol B, Morange S, Loundoun A, et al. A randomized trial of saline hydration to prevent contrast nephropathy in chronic renal failure patients. Nephrol Dial Transplant 2006;21:2120–6.

33. Briguori C, Visconti G, Focaccio A, et al, REMEDIAL II Investigators. Renal Insufficiency After Contrast Media Administration Trial II (REMEDIAL II): RenalGuard system in high-risk patients for contrast-induced acute kidney injury. Circulation 2011;124:1260–9.

34. Marenzi G, Ferrari C, Marana I, et al. Prevention of contrast nephropathy by furosemide with matched hydration: the MYTHOS (Induced Diuresis With Matched Hydration Compared to Standard Hydration for Contrast Induced Nephropathy Prevention) trial. JACC Cardiovasc Interv 2012;5:90–7.

35. Briguori C, Visconti G, Ricciardelli B, et al, REMEDIAL II Investigators. Renal Insufficiency Following Contrast Media Administration Trial II (REMEDIAL II): RenalGuard system in high-risk patients for contrast-induced acute kidney injury: rationale and design. EuroIntervention 2011;6:1117–22,. 1117.

36. Stone GW, Vora K, Schindler J, et al. Systemic hypothermia to prevent radiocontrast nephropathy (from the COOL-RCN randomized trial). Am J Cardiol 2011;108:741–6.

37. Talati S, Kirtane AJ, Hassanin A, et al. Direct infusion of fenoldopam into the renal arteries to protect against contrast-induced nephropathy in patients at increased risk. Clin Exp Pharmacol Physiol 2012;39:506–9.

38. Babsky A, Hekmatyar S, Wehrli S, et al. Influence of ischemic preconditioning on intracellular sodium, pH, and cellular energy status in isolated perfused heart. Exp Biol Med (Maywood) 2002;227:520–8.

39. Miura T, Tanno M. The mPTP and its regulatory proteins: final common targets of signalling pathways for protection against necrosis. Cardiovasc Res 2012;94:181–9.

40. Peart JN, Headrick JP. Clinical cardioprotection and the value of conditioning responses. Am J Physiol Heart Circ Physiol 2009;296:H1705–20.

41. Sun J, Aponte AM, Kohr MJ, et al. Essential role of nitric oxide in acute ischemic preconditioning: S-nitros(yl)ation versus sGC/cGMP/PKG signaling? Free Radic Biol Med 2013;54:105–12.

42. Serviddio G, Di Venosa N, Federici A, et al. Brief hypoxia before normoxic reperfusion (postconditioning) protects the heart against ischemia-reperfusion injury by preventing mitochondria peroxyde production and glutathione depletion. FASEB J 2005;19:354–61.

43. Konstantinov IE, Arab S, Li J, et al. The remote ischemic preconditioning stimulus modifies gene expression in mouse myocardium. J Thorac Cardiovasc Surg 2005;130:1326–32.

44. Venugopal V, Laing CM, Ludman A, et al. Effect of remote ischemic preconditioning on acute kidney injury in nondiabetic patients undergoing coronary artery bypass graft surgery: a secondary analysis of 2 small randomized trials. Am J Kidney Dis 2010;56:1043–9.

45. Zimmerman RF, Ezeanuna PU, Kane JC, et al. Ischemic preconditioning at a remote site prevents acute kidney injury in patients following cardiac surgery. Kidney Int 2011;80:861–7.

46. Walsh SR, Sadat U, Boyle JR, et al. Remote ischemic preconditioning for renal protection during elective open infrarenal abdominal aortic aneurysm repair: randomized controlled trial. Vasc Endovascular Surg 2010;44:334–40.

47. Choi YS, Shim JK, Kim JC, et al. Effect of remote ischemic preconditioning on renal dysfunction after complex valvular heart surgery: a randomized controlled trial. J Thorac Cardiovasc Surg 2011;142:148–54.

48. Li L, Li G, Yu C, et al. The role of remote ischemic preconditioning on postoperative kidney injury in patients undergoing cardiac and vascular interventions: a meta-analysis. J Cardiothorac Surg 2013;8:43.

49. Er F, Nia AM, Dopp H, et al. Ischemic preconditioning for prevention of contrast medium-induced nephropathy: randomized pilot RenPro Trial (Renal Protection Trial). Circulation 2012;126:296–303.

50. Deftereos S, Giannopoulos G, Tzalamouras V, et al. Renoprotective effect of remote ischemic postconditioning by intermittent balloon inflations in patients undergoing percutaneous coronary intervention. J Am Coll Cardiol 2013;61:1949–55.

A Practical Approach to Preventing Renal Complications in the Catheterization Laboratory

 CrossMark

Michael Howe, MD[a],*, Hitinder S. Gurm, MD[b]

KEYWORDS

- Radiocontrast • Nephropathy • Kidney • Hydration • Catheterization

KEY POINTS

- Kidney injury associated with cardiac catheterization occurs infrequently but may have serious and prolonged complications.
- Patients at risk for renal complications may be identified by risk factors and risk-prediction models.
- Institutions should follow a standardized approach to minimize the risk of contrast injury in all patients.
- The 3 key elements of this approach are:
  - Ensuring appropriate hydration before, during, and after the procedure
  - Preprocedural assessment of glomerular filtration rate and appropriate dosing of contrast media
  - Preferentially using iso-osmolar contrast or low-osmolar contrast media that have been associated with lower risk of renal complications
- High-dose statin preloading may be potentially beneficial in reducing the risk of contrast injury, and should be considered in all patients undergoing percutaneous coronary intervention given the other benefits of statin therapy in this patient population.

BACKGROUND

Kidney injury following cardiac catheterization may occur for several reasons, including radiocontrast exposure, atheroembolism, or hypotension and renal hypoperfusion. The rates of acute kidney injury (AKI) following cardiac catheterization are variably reported in the literature depending on the definition used, type of contrast media, and patient subset, typically ranging from as low as 1% to as high as 20% of cases.[1-3] When it does occur, AKI can lead to accumulation of metabolic byproducts, fluid retention, electrolyte and acid-base abnormalities, and a high correlation with death both in the hospital and following discharge.[4-6] In a cohort analysis of more than 16,000 patients undergoing radiocontrast procedures, the risk of developing postprocedure AKI was less than 2%; those who did develop AKI, however, were more than 5 times more likely to die in the hospital.[7]

AKI, as defined by the international Kidney Disease: Improving Global Outcomes (KDIGO) initiative, is either an increase in serum creatinine by 0.3 mg/dL or more (≥26.5 μmol/L) within 48 hours,

---

The authors have nothing to disclose.

[a] Division of Cardiovascular Medicine, Department of Internal Medicine, Frankel Cardiovascular Center, University of Michigan Health System, 1500 East Medical Center Drive, Ann Arbor, MI 48109-5869, USA;
[b] Division of Cardiovascular Medicine, Department of Internal Medicine, Frankel Cardiovascular Center, University of Michigan Health System, University of Michigan Cardiovascular Center, 1500 East Medical Center Drive, 2A394, Ann Arbor, MI 48109-5869, USA
* Corresponding author.
E-mail address: michowe@med.umich.edu

Intervent Cardiol Clin 3 (2014) 429–439
http://dx.doi.org/10.1016/j.iccl.2014.03.011

interventional.theclinics.com

an increase in serum creatinine to greater than 1.5 times baseline within 7 days, or urine volume of less than 0.5 mL/kg/h for 6 hours.[8] Of note, the studies that have established the poor outcome in association with AKI among patients undergoing cardiac procedures have generally used an absolute increase in serum creatinine of 0.5 mg/dL or greater to define AKI. There has been considerable investigation into strategies to mitigate the development of AKI following cardiac catheterization, with the majority focused on the prevention of contrast-induced nephropathy (CIN).

MECHANISM AND CLINICAL MANIFESTATIONS

The details of the mechanism and pathophysiology of CIN are discussed at greater length elsewhere in this issue by Geenen and colleagues. In brief, CIN, despite its association with increased mortality, is generally a reversible process. Serum creatinine levels typically increase 24 to 48 hours after radiocontrast exposure, with a peak at 4 to 5 days before return to baseline levels at 7 to 10 days.[9] The need for dialysis following CIN appears to be low, and varies depending on underlying risk factors. When the need for dialysis does occur, however, it portends a grim prognosis. A single-center study found an in-hospital mortality of more than 35% for patients who developed AKI requiring dialysis following coronary intervention, with a 2-year survival rate of 19%.[4] The extrarenal manifestations and symptoms of CIN are relatively few, and the renal failure is typically nonoliguric.[10] Laboratory abnormalities including electrolyte and acid-base disturbances are reflective of decreased renal clearance, and urinalysis may show nonspecific casts suggestive of tubular injury.[11]

CIN may occur through both renal vasoconstriction and direct tubular injury, although the exact mechanism remains unclear. Studies in both animal and human models have suggested a complex interplay between vasodilator and vasoconstrictor influences including nitric oxide, prostaglandin, and endothelin systems, in addition to generated reactive oxygen species and direct cytotoxic properties of contrast medium itself.[10,12] Investigation into these mechanisms has suggested several possible targets for prevention or mitigation of CIN, although clinical adaptation has been limited.

RISK FACTORS AND PREDICTION MODELS

Kidney injury following cardiac catheterization has been clearly associated with multiple patient-related and procedure-related risk factors, with the risk increasing additively along with the number of risk factors.[13] Preexisting renal insufficiency, defined as a serum creatinine greater than 1.5 mg/dL or estimated glomerular filtration rate (eGFR) less than 60 mL/min/1.73 m^2 is the strongest baseline predictor of CIN following percutaneous coronary intervention (PCI) according to a large data set reported by Mehran and colleagues,[14] with higher risk associated with more severe baseline renal dysfunction.[3] Other prominent risk factors for the development of CIN include New York Heart Association (NYHA) class III to IV congestive heart failure, advanced age, and history of diabetes mellitus with associated renal insufficiency.[12] In elderly cohorts older than 65 years, women appear to be at increased risk for development of CIN following cardiac catheterization in comparison with men.[2]

These risk factors have been assimilated into several different risk-prediction models that have sought to identify patients at risk for developing CIN. In 2004, Mehran and colleagues[14] published a risk score based on 8 different patient-related and procedure-related risk factors. In this model, risk factors of hypotension, necessity of intra-aortic balloon pump (IABP), NYHA class III to IV congestive heart failure, age older than 75 years, anemia, diabetes, contrast volume, and preprocedure renal function were weighted into 4 quartiles of increasing risk of developing CIN or requiring dialysis with a c-statistic of 0.67. However, the poor discrimination of this model and the inclusion of procedural variables limit the utility of this risk score for preprocedural risk stratification.

A more contemporary risk model for the development of renal complications in patients undergoing PCI was proposed in 2013; developed from 15 different influential variables associated with the patient's history, presentation, and preprocedure laboratory assessments. The patient characteristics shown in **Box 1** are factored into a weighted algorithm that stratifies patients into low (<1%), intermediate (1%–7%), and high (>7%) risk groups based on the risk of CIN.[15] This model was validated in a cohort of patients undergoing PCI and requires a computer for calculation (https://bmc2.org/calculators/cin); however, it appears to be statistically superior, with an area under the curve of 0.839, and has the added the benefit of being composed solely of preprocedural variables.

At present, however, neither the 2012 American College of Cardiology Foundation/Society for Cardiovascular Angiography and Interventions (ACCF/SCAI) nor the KDIGO guidelines have made formal recommendations for preprocedure risk-algorithm utilization other than establishing those at risk via eGFR.[8,16] The suggested protocol

Box 1
Patient and procedural characteristics included in the BMC2 risk model

Patient presentation

   PCI indication

   PCI status

   CAD presentation

   Cardiogenic shock

   Heart failure within 2 weeks

   Pre-PCI left ventricular ejection fraction

Clinical history

   Diabetes mellitus/diabetes therapy

Patient characteristics

   Age, years

   Weight, kg

   Height, cm

Preprocedural laboratory assessments

   Creatinine kinase MB

   Serum creatinine

   Hemoglobin

   Troponin I

   Troponin T

Abbreviations: BMC2, The Blue Cross Blue Shield of Michigan Cardiovascular Consortium; CAD, coronary artery disease; PCI, percutaneous coronary intervention.
   From Gurm HS, Seth M, Kooiman J, et al. A novel tool for reliable and accurate prediction of renal complications in patients undergoing percutaneous coronary intervention. J Am Coll Cardiol 2013;61:2244; with permission.

Box 2
2012 ACCF/SCAI suggested protocol for reducing the incidence of contrast-associated nephropathy

Identify risks

   Highest risk: eGFR less than 60 mL/min/1.73 m^2

   Diabetes

Manage medications

   Hold nephrotoxic drugs (eg, NSAIDs)

Manage intravascular volume

   Hydrate with either normal saline or sodium bicarbonate (either acceptable)

   Hydrate with 1.0 to 1.5 mL/kg/min for 3 to 12 hours before and 6 to 12 hours after

Radiographic contrast

   Minimize contrast volume

   Use either low-osmolar or iso-osmolar contrast

Follow-up data

   Obtain 48-hour creatinine

Abbreviations: eGFR, estimated glomerular filtration rate; NSAIDs, nonsteroidal anti-inflammatory drugs.
   From Bashore TM, Balter S, Barac A, et al. 2012 American College of Cardiology Foundation/Society for Cardiovascular Angiography and Interventions expert consensus document on cardiac catheterization laboratory standards update: a report of the American College of Cardiology Foundation Task Force on Expert Consensus documents developed in collaboration with the Society of Thoracic Surgeons and Society for Vascular Medicine. J Am Coll Cardiol 2012;59:2264; with permission.

by the ACCF/SCAI Expert Consensus Document on Cardiac Catheterization Laboratory Standards for minimizing CIN is shown in **Box 2.** The KDIGO document only recommends assessment of risk and screening for preexisting renal impairment before intravascular contrast exposure.

CONTRAST MEDIA

Significant improvements in the safety profile of radiocontrast agents used during cardiac catheterization have occurred with the development of low-osmolar (iohexol, iopamidol, iopromide) and newer iso-osmolar (iodixanol, iotrolan) compounds. First-generation hyperosmolar agents have been associated with increased risk for CIN in comparison with newer agents.[17,18] Likewise, there may be a lower risk of CIN with iso-osmolar

agents compared with certain low-osmolar agents, especially in certain subgroups such as patients with chronic kidney disease (CKD),[19,20] although a more recent meta-analysis found no significant difference in the rates of CIN between the iso-osmolar agent iodixanol and a pool of low-osmolar agents.[21] Guidelines from the 2012 ACCF/SCAI Expert Consensus Document on Cardiac Catheterization Laboratory Standards reflect this, recommending the use of either low-osmolar or iso-osmolar agents without differentiation.[16]

   It is also recognized that higher volumes of radiocontrast administration are associated with an increased risk of CIN,[4,22] especially in patients with multiple risk factors.[6] The maximal acceptable contrast dose (MACD) has been proposed as a tool to guide contrast administration volumes and identify a contrast limit in patients with renal disease.[23] The MACD is calculated using the formula maximum dose = 5 mL × (body weight in kg)/(serum creatinine in mg/dL), and has been validated to help reduce the rate of CIN in high-risk patients.[6] Newer prediction models have used the calculated creatinine clearance (CCC) to define the safe volume of radiocontrast; a strategy that appears to be superior to the MACD formula and clearly emphasizes the effect of higher contrast doses.[24,25] Using a cohort of patients undergoing PCI from the Blue Cross Blue Shield of Michigan Cardiovascular Consortium (BMC2) registry, a ratio of contrast dose to CCC of greater than 2 approached significance for risk of CIN, whereas a ratio of greater than 3 yielded a significant and substantial increase in the risk of developing CIN.[24]

Measures to reduce contrast volume should be considered in all patients, as should a strategy of keeping the contrast dose as low as possible. Forgoing left ventriculography and aortography can yield substantial reductions in contrast dose. The use of biplane coronary angiography can also be especially helpful in reducing the volume of contrast required during diagnostic catheterization.

Catheter selection, such as using a 6F guide catheter instead of a 7F or 8F system when the technicalities of the procedure allow, can also help significantly reduce the volume of contrast administered during the operation. In patients undergoing PCI, the use of 6F guide catheters has been associated with lower rates of postprocedure nephropathy in addition to fewer vascular complications and lower mortality, especially when compared with larger 8F guide catheters.[26]

Intravascular ultrasonography (IVUS) may be helpful in the assessment of lesion length and diameter as a means of minimizing contrast volume during PCI, and has been used in cases with very little contrast exposure.[27] Likewise, newer technologies such as the GuideLiner catheter (Vascular Solutions, Minneapolis, MN) may also be used as a means of subselecting the artery of interest during PCI to minimize contrast administration while allowing adequate visualization of the culprit lesion (ie, selective left circumflex angiography).[28]

Another possible solution to minimizing contrast exposure is the use of automated contrast injection systems. These devices offer a theoretical advantage over manual hand injections in terms of reduction in the volume of contrast delivered during angiography,[29,30] with some studies suggesting a decreased incidence of CIN.[31,32] However, more recent studies have failed to confirm a significant reduction in the rates of renal complications (CIN or need for dialysis) among centers that use automated contrast injection systems,[33,34] and at present seem to offer no clear benefit over careful and moderated hand-based contrast administration.

At times, however, with large impending contrast loads for complex interventions in patients with CKD or multiple CIN risk factors, it may be beneficial to divide the contrast load between staged procedures.[23] Given the risk of repeat contrast exposure within close temporal proximity,[35] a 2006 CIN Consensus Working Panel recommended 2 weeks be allowed between staged procedures to allow renal recovery.[36]

PREVENTION STRATEGIES

Beyond limiting exposure to contrast agents, multiple agents and periprocedural interventions have been suggested as strategies for reducing the risk of renal complications following cardiac catheterization. Perhaps the most widely and frequently used approach is intravenous volume expansion. With radiocontrast-induced vasoconstriction leading to renal medullary ischemia[37] implicated in the mechanism of kidney injury, oral and intravenous hydration both have been explored as possible preventive approaches. Initial investigation into the use of diuretics as a means of decreasing the rate of CIN have not borne out significant benefit, and in fact appear to show an increase in the incidence of CIN when compared with intravenous hydration.[38,39] Although the recent, small MYTHOS (Induced Diuresis With Matched Hydration Compared with Standard Hydration for Contrast Induced Nephropathy Prevention) trial did find a reduction in the incidence of CIN in CKD patients treated with diuretic-induced high urine output with matched hydration,[40] this strategy has not been incorporated into major guideline recommendations[8,16] and is not considered standard practice.

The data supporting volume expansion as a means of mitigating the renal effects of radiocontrast exposure are clearer, although debate remains regarding the ideal fluid, rate, and duration.[41,42] In a randomized study of more than 1600 patients undergoing coronary angioplasty, isotonic (0.9% saline) was found to be superior to half-tonic (0.45% NaCl with 5% glucose) in the prevention of kidney injury.[43] This finding has led to a recommendation for preferential use of isotonic saline in recent ACCF/SCAI guidelines,[16] although there is also evidence suggesting a role of sodium bicarbonate infusion before contrast exposure.

In theory, alkalinization of tubular fluid via hydration with sodium bicarbonate may protect against the nephrotoxic effects of oxygen free radicals associated with contrast exposure.[44] A randomized trial from Merten and colleagues[45] in 2004 found that in 119 patients with normal renal function undergoing radiocontrast examinations, hydration with sodium bicarbonate for 1 hour before contrast and continuing for 6 hours after contrast exposure was more effective than pretreatment with sodium chloride in the prevention of CIN. Similar results were seen in a population at moderate risk of CIN undergoing coronary angiography, with a significant reduction of 71% in the risk of CIN while using sodium bicarbonate compared with normal saline, albeit with a longer pretreatment duration of 6 hours before contrast exposure.[46] Both studies, however, had small sample sizes, and a 2010 meta-analysis demonstrated wide variation among trials, with only borderline statistical significance for the beneficial effect of sodium bicarbonate in the prevention of CIN; this effect, however, was strongest in urgent coronary angiography procedures.[47] Owing to inconsistent data and the increased burden of bicarbonate preparation, current recommendations do not support a preference for the use of bicarbonate over normal saline as a means of volume expansion.[8]

Several trials have also explored the role of acetylcysteine as an adjuvant therapy in the prevention of CIN. As an antioxidant, acetylcysteine has been evaluated both alone and in combination with sodium chloride and sodium bicarbonate hydration before contrast exposure. An initial study of 83 patients found that acetylcysteine in combination with 0.45% normal saline was superior to placebo and saline in the prevention of CIN following contrast exposure on computed tomography scanning.[48] Since then, however, significant heterogeneity has been reported. Whereas some trials, including the RENO Study[49] and the REMEDIAL Trial,[50] have observed some reduction in the rate of CIN following administration of acetylcysteine in combination with sodium bicarbonate, others have found no benefit from the addition of acetylcysteine.[46] The recently published large, randomized ACT (Acetylcysteine for the prevention of Contrast-induced nephropathy Trial) found no benefit of prophylactic administration of acetylcysteine in the reduction of CIN or secondary end points of all-cause mortality or need for dialysis at 30 days.[51] Likewise, a recent review of patients undergoing PCI from the BMC2 multicenter cohort also found no difference in outcomes in patients treated with acetylcysteine in a real-world practice setting,[52] and at present it is no longer recommended.[16]

Investigation into other medical prevention strategies has been active and ongoing for many years, and more recently the use of high-dose statin therapy as a means of mitigating inflammatory and oxidative stress associated with radiocontrast exposure has been suggested. Although there are no formal recommendations at this time for routine statin administration before contrast exposure, there are both observational and randomized data suggesting benefit.[53–56] In the recently published Protective Effect of Rosuvastatin and Antiplatelet Therapy on Contrast-Induced Acute Kidney Injury and Myocardial Damage in Patients with Acute Coronary Syndrome (PRATO-ACS) study, treatment of statin-naïve ACS patients undergoing PCI with high-dose rosuvastatin was associated with significantly lower rates of CIN and improved cardiovascular outcomes.[57] Given the known benefits of statin therapy in both stable and unstable coronary artery disease, it is reasonable to include pretreatment with high-dose statins for both renoprotective and cardioprotective purposes in this patient population.

Avoidance of nephrotoxic medication, when possible, may also have a role in minimizing renal complications following catheterization. Nephrotoxic medications such as nonsteroidal anti-inflammatory drugs (NSAIDs) should be stopped, if possible, before catheterization.[8] Although there is an association between the use of high-dose metformin and the development of lactic acidosis,[58] metformin itself is not directly nephrotoxic, and there are no data regarding an association between cardiac catheterization and metformin-associated lactic acidosis.[59,60] Despite this, a policy of holding metformin before contrast exposure remains prominent in the protocols of many catheterization laboratories. This policy is reiterated in the 2012 ACCF/SCAI Cardiac Catheterization Laboratory Standards document, which recommends holding metformin the day of the procedure and for at least 48 hours afterward until a normal creatinine has been documented,[16] although recent European Society of Cardiology guidelines advocate careful monitoring of renal function after the procedure and holding metformin for 48 hours only if it deteriorates.[61]

Retrospective data suggest a risk association between preoperative use of angiotensin-converting enzyme (ACE) inhibitors or angiotensin-receptor blocking medications and development of CIN.[62,63] However, other reports suggest a possible renoprotective role of these medications,[64] and there is no evidence that withholding these medications alone before catheterization decreases the incidence of CIN.[65] At present there is no evidence to suggest that these medications should be stopped before catheterization in the setting of stable renal function. Likewise, if a patient is not already on an ACE inhibitor or angiotensin-receptor blocker, there is no indication for starting one before radiocontrast exposure.

Routine hemofiltration and hemodialysis have been evaluated as periprocedural means of removing the offending radiocontrast agent in those patients at high risk for development of CIN, although a 2012 meta-analysis found no significant benefit over standard medical therapy, and neither is routinely recommended.[66]

TIMING OF TREATMENT

While there is clear benefit to intravenous hydration and volume expansion as a means of mitigating renal injury during cardiac catheterization, the timing of these regimens, especially in the setting of emergency procedures for unstable coronary syndromes, has also been the source of much investigation.

When timing allows, preprocedure hydration seems to be superior to hydration during the procedure alone.[67] However, there is no direct evidence guiding the optimal starting time for hydration. It appears that longer courses of hydration, such as overnight[68] or 20 hours,[69] are not superior to bolus or shorter courses of hydration. Several studies have evaluated hydration strategies using 12-hour protocols, which has led some investigators to recommend hydration with 1 mL/kg/h isotonic saline for 12 hours before and 12 hours after radiocontrast administration, with an abbreviated regimen of 3 mL/kg/h for 1 hour before and 6 hours after a more urgent procedure.[42] A 2006 CIN Consensus Working Panel recommended an optimal protocol of 1 to 1.5 mL/kg/h intravenous isotonic saline for 3 to 12 hours before and 6 to 24 hours after radiocontrast exposure.[70] Current ACCF/SCAI guidelines recommend preprocedure hydration with either normal saline or sodium bicarbonate, 1.0 to 1.5 mL/kg/min for 3 to 12 hours before and 6 to 12 hours after the procedure.[16]

The recently reported results of the POSEIDON (Prevention of Contrast Renal Injury with Different Hydration Strategies) trial, announced in late 2012, evaluated the use of left ventricular end-diastolic pressure (LVEDP)-guided sliding-scale hydration for a personalized rate of periprocedure hydration. This single-center study included 396 patients with eGFR less than 60 mL/min/1.73 m^2 undergoing coronary angiography and/or PCI, who were randomized to a standard hydration protocol with 0.9% normal saline at 3 mL/kg for 1 hour preprocedure followed by 1.5 mL/kg/h during the procedure and continued for 4 hours postprocedure, or an LVEDP-guided strategy with 0.9%

normal saline at 3 mL/kg for 1 hour preprocedure and continued periprocedure hydration at a rate determined by LVEDP (LVEDP <13 then 5 mL/kg/h, LVEDP 13–18 then 3 mL/kg/h, or LVEDP >18 then 1.5 mL/kg/h) continuing for 4 hours postprocedure. The LVEDP-guided hydration group received higher volumes of intravenous hydration overall than the standard hydration group, with a significant 59% relative reduction and 10% absolute reduction in the incidence of CIN.[71] There were no differences between groups in terms of the number of patients who required termination of intravenous hydration, in most cases for shortness of breath.

PRACTICAL CONSIDERATIONS

There is extensive heterogeneity of data regarding the prevention of renal complications in the catheterization laboratory, and it can be challenging to apply this information to a broad patient population with significant differences in risk factors, baseline renal function, and procedure urgency. In general, practical consideration must be applied on an individual case-level basis so as not to delay an emergent procedure or rush hastily into a case with a negative outcome that could have been prevented. From a practical perspective, the emphasis should be on ensuring adequate preprocedure and periprocedure hydration with either normal saline or sodium bicarbonate. Given the data already presented herein and the lack of clear superiority of one contrast agent over another, the authors recommend establishing a catheterization laboratory protocol with either agent and applying this strategy uniformly across all patients at risk.

Likewise, nephrotoxic medications including NSAIDs and aminoglycosides (if possible) should be withheld before contrast administration in patients at increased risk of CIN. High-dose statin therapy should be initiated before catheterization both for renoprotective purposes and because of its established atherosclerotic benefits in this patient population.

An algorithmic approach, illustrated in **Fig. 1**, suggests a strategy for risk assessment, monitoring, and intervention during cardiac catheterization. An initial risk assessment should be undertaken before all nonemergent cases; a practical approach would favor the use of the model proposed by Gurm and colleagues[15] over the Mehran model,[14] because it comprises readily available preprocedure variables. This model should be incorporated, along with a confirmation of the eGFR and contrast-dose thresholds, into the preprocedure "time-out" undertaken in the catheterization laboratory before procedure

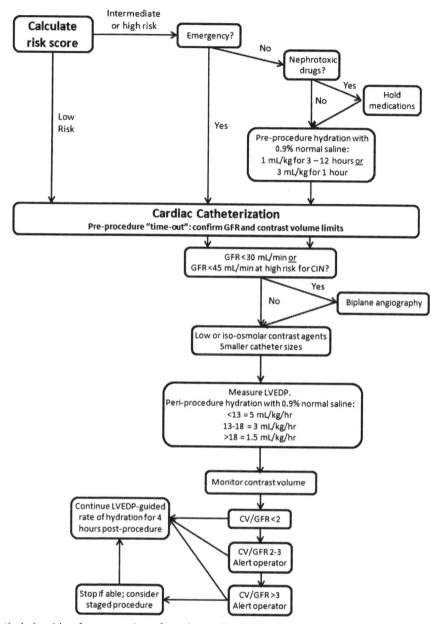

Fig. 1. Practical algorithm for prevention of renal complications in the cardiac catheterization laboratory. Risk-score calculator is online (https://bmc2.org/calculators/cin) and is described by Gurm and colleagues.[15] Intermediate or high risk is defined as ≥1% chance of CIN. CIN, contrast-induced nephropathy; CV, contrast volume; GFR, glomerular filtration rate; LVEDP, left ventricular end-diastolic pressure.

initiation, with the goal of ensuring that all team members are aware of the renal risks and limits to contrast utilization. Following risk and urgency stratification, preprocedure hydration should be administered to patients at intermediate or high risk of CIN. Periprocedure and postprocedure hydration should continue at a rate guided by LVEDP as outlined in the POSEIDON trial.[71]

During the procedure, judicious use of biplane cineangiography, smaller-gauge diagnostic and guide catheters, and low-osmolar or iso-osmolar contrast agents should be applied where feasible in patients at risk. Finally, laboratory staff should continuously monitor the volume of contrast used during the case, with verbal alerts provided to the operator when contrast volume to eGFR ratios of 2 and 3 are met or exceeded. When necessary and feasible, staged procedures should be considered to minimize and divide contrast exposures. Following the procedure, hydration should be continued as tolerated and guided by the pre-procedure renal function and volume status, with a follow-up assessment of renal function within 48 hours. Elevation in serum creatinine above baseline and development of AKI following cardiac catheterization should be managed with further hydration and volume optimization, in addition to continued avoidance of nephrotoxic medications. Progressive renal dysfunction should be managed in consultation with a nephrologist when available.

Procedures can be performed using extremely low volumes of contrast when care and time are taken to minimize waste. An example by Nayak and colleagues[72] describes the use of less than 15 mL of contrast during coronary angiography and PCI through a combination of biplane cinean-giography, small (3 mL) contrast syringes for stricter control, higher angiography frame rates, minimal "tests" and "puffs," and increased utiliza-tion of IVUS for assessment of lesion characteris-tics. Though an extreme example, this does highlight the power of combining several of these preventive strategies. The authors routinely use such strategies, and have been successful at completing complex procedures with minimal contrast volume.

SUMMARY

Renal complications following cardiac catheteriza-tion occur infrequently, but can have significant ef-fects on morbidity and mortality. A variety of mechanisms may account for kidney injury, some of which can be a direct result of the ongoing car-diac disorder. A significant amount of effort has been invested in the identification and treatment of patients at increased risk for renal complica-tions, with variable results. Perhaps the most beneficial, and easily applicable, intervention is minimizing the amount of radiocontrast dye used during the case. Additional renal protection may be afforded by volume expansion with intravenous hydration before, during, and after the catheteriza-tion, with administration rates guided by the pa-tient's intravascular volume status and clinical stability. Further progress continues toward safer radiocontrast agents, catheterization techniques, and therapeutic preventive strategies to minimize renal injury following angiographic procedures.

REFERENCES

1. Bartholomew BA, Harjai KJ, Dukkipati S, et al. Impact of nephropathy after percutaneous coro-nary intervention and a method for risk stratifica-tion. Am J Cardiol 2004;93:1515–9.

2. Sidhu RB, Brown JR, Robb JF, et al. Interaction of gender and age on post cardiac catheterization contrast-induced acute kidney injury. Am J Cardiol 2008;102:1482–6.

3. Rihal CS, Textor SC, Grill DE, et al. Incidence and prognostic importance of acute renal failure after percutaneous coronary intervention. Circulation 2002;105:2259–64.

4. McCullough PA, Wolyn R, Rocher LL, et al. Acute renal failure after coronary intervention: incidence, risk factors, and relationship to mortality. Am J Med 1997;103:368–75.

5. Gupta R, Gurm HS, Bhatt DL, et al. Renal failure after percutaneous coronary intervention is associ-ated with high mortality. Catheter Cardiovasc Interv 2005;64:442–8.

6. Freeman RV, O'Donnell M, Share D, et al. Nephrop-athy requiring dialysis after percutaneous coronary intervention and the critical role of an adjusted contrast dose. Am J Cardiol 2002;90:1068–73.

7. Levy EM, Viscoli CM, Horwitz RI. The effect of acute renal failure on mortality. A cohort analysis. JAMA 1996;275:1489–94.

8. Kidney Disease: Improving Global Outcomes (KDIGO) Acute Kidney Injury Work Group. KDIGO clinical practice guideline for acute kidney injury. Kidney Int 2012;2:1–138.

9. Solomon R. Contrast-medium-induced acute renal failure. Kidney Int 1998;53:230–42.

10. Kaul A, Sharma RK, Tripathi R, et al. Spectrum of community-acquired acute kidney injury in India: a retrospective study. Saudi J Kidney Dis Transpl 2012;23:619–28.

11. Gleeson TG, Bulugahapitiya S. Contrast-induced nephropathy. AJR Am J Roentgenol 2004;183:1673–89.

12. Wong PC, Li Z, Guo J, et al. Pathophysiology of contrast-induced nephropathy. Int J Cardiol 2012;158:186–92.

13. Bartorelli AL, Marenzi G. Contrast-induced nephro-pathy. J Interv Cardiol 2008;21:74–85.

14. Mehran R, Aymong ED, Nikolsky E, et al. A simple risk score for prediction of contrast-induced neph-ropathy after percutaneous coronary intervention: development and initial validation. J Am Coll Car-diol 2004;44:1393–9.

15. Gurm HS, Seth M, Kooiman J, et al. A novel tool for reliable and accurate prediction of renal complica-tions in patients undergoing percutaneous coro-nary intervention. J Am Coll Cardiol 2013;61:2242–8.

16. Bashore TM, Balter S, Barac A, et al. 2012 American College of Cardiology Foundation/Society for Car-diovascular Angiography and Interventions expert consensus document on cardiac catheterization laboratory standards update: a report of the American College of Cardiology Foundation Task

Force on Expert Consensus documents developed in collaboration with the Society of Thoracic Surgeons and Society for Vascular Medicine. J Am Coll Cardiol 2012;59:2221–305.

17. Barrett BJ, Carlisle EJ. Metaanalysis of the relative nephrotoxicity of high- and low-osmolality iodinated contrast media. Radiology 1993;188:171–8.

18. Rudnick MR, Goldfarb S, Wexler L, et al. Nephrotoxicity of ionic and nonionic contrast media in 1196 patients: a randomized trial. The Iohexol Cooperative Study. Kidney Int 1995;47:254–61.

19. McCullough PA, Bertrand ME, Brinker JA, et al. A meta-analysis of the renal safety of isosmolar iodixanol compared with low-osmolar contrast media. J Am Coll Cardiol 2006;48:692–9.

20. Aspelin P, Aubry P, Fransson SG, et al. Nephrotoxic effects in high-risk patients undergoing angiography. N Engl J Med 2003;348:491–9.

21. Reed M, Meier P, Tamhane UU, et al. The relative renal safety of iodixanol compared with low-osmolar contrast media: a meta-analysis of randomized controlled trials. JACC Cardiovasc Interv 2009;2:645–54.

22. Brown JR, Robb JF, Block CA, et al. Does safe dosing of iodinated contrast prevent contrast-induced acute kidney injury? Circ Cardiovasc Interv 2010;3:346–50.

23. Cigarroa RG, Lange RA, Williams RH, et al. Dosing of contrast material to prevent contrast nephropathy in patients with renal disease. Am J Med 1989;86:649–52.

24. Gurm HS, Dixon SR, Smith DE, et al. Renal function-based contrast dosing to define safe limits of radiographic contrast media in patients undergoing percutaneous coronary interventions. J Am Coll Cardiol 2011;58:907–14.

25. Laskey WK, Jenkins C, Selzer F, et al. Volume-to-creatinine clearance ratio: a pharmacokinetically based risk factor for prediction of early creatinine increase after percutaneous coronary intervention. J Am Coll Cardiol 2007;50:584–90.

26. Grossman PM, Gurm HS, McNamara R, et al. Percutaneous coronary intervention complications and guide catheter size: bigger is not better. JACC Cardiovasc Interv 2009;2:636–44.

27. Ogata N, Matsukage T, Toda E, et al. Intravascular ultrasound-guided percutaneous coronary interventions with minimum contrast volume for prevention of the radiocontrast-induced nephropathy: report of two cases. Cardiovasc Interv Ther 2011; 26:83–8.

28. Tunuguntla A, Daneault B, Kirtane AJ. Novel use of the GuideLiner catheter to minimize contrast use during PCI in a patient with chronic kidney disease. Catheter Cardiovasc Interv 2012;80:453–5.

29. Chahoud G, Khoukaz S, El-Shafei A, et al. Randomized comparison of coronary angiography using 4F catheters: 4F manual versus "Acisted" power injection technique. Catheter Cardiovasc Interv 2001;53:221–4.

30. Anne G, Gruberg L, Huber A, et al. Traditional versus automated injection contrast system in diagnostic and percutaneous coronary interventional procedures: comparison of the contrast volume delivered. J Invasive Cardiol 2004;16:360–2.

31. Call J, Sacrinty M, Applegate R, et al. Automated contrast injection in contemporary practice during cardiac catheterization and PCI: effects on contrast-induced nephropathy. J Invasive Cardiol 2006;18:469–74.

32. Godley RW 2nd, Joshi K, Breall JA. A comparison of the use of traditional hand injection versus automated contrast injectors during cardiac catheterization. J Invasive Cardiol 2012;24:628–30.

33. Hwang JR, D'Alfonso S, Kostuk WJ, et al. Contrast volume use in manual vs automated contrast injection systems for diagnostic coronary angiography and percutaneous coronary interventions. Can J Cardiol 2013;29:372–6.

34. Gurm HS, Smith D, Share D, et al. Impact of automated contrast injector systems on contrast use and contrast-associated complications in patients undergoing percutaneous coronary interventions. JACC Cardiovasc Interv 2013;6:399–405.

35. Taliercio CP, Vlietstra RE, Fisher LD, et al. Risks for renal dysfunction with cardiac angiography. Ann Intern Med 1986;104:501–4.

36. Davidson C, Stacul F, McCullough PA, et al. Contrast medium use. Am J Cardiol 2006;98: 42K–58K.

37. Heyman SN, Brezis M, Epstein FH, et al. Early renal medullary hypoxic injury from radiocontrast and indomethacin. Kidney Int 1991;40:632–42.

38. Solomon R, Werner C, Mann D, et al. Effects of saline, mannitol, and furosemide to prevent acute decreases in renal function induced by radiocontrast agents. N Engl J Med 1994;331:1416–20.

39. Majumdar SR, Kjellstrand CM, Tymchak WJ, et al. Forced euvolemic diuresis with mannitol and furosemide for prevention of contrast-induced nephropathy in patients with CKD undergoing coronary angiography: a randomized controlled trial. Am J Kidney Dis 2009;54:602–9.

40. Marenzi G, Ferrari C, Marana I, et al. Prevention of contrast nephropathy by furosemide with matched hydration: the MYTHOS (Induced Diuresis With Matched Hydration Compared to Standard Hydration for Contrast Induced Nephropathy Prevention) trial. JACC Cardiovasc Interv 2012;5:90–7.

41. Trivedi HS, Moore H, Nasr S, et al. A randomized prospective trial to assess the role of saline hydration on the development of contrast nephrotoxicity. Nephron Clin Pract 2003;93:C29–34.

42. Weisbord SD, Palevsky PM. Prevention of contrast-induced nephropathy with volume expansion. Clin J Am Soc Nephrol 2008;3:273–80.

43. Mueller C, Buerkle G, Buettner HJ, et al. Prevention of contrast media-associated nephropathy: randomized comparison of 2 hydration regimens in 1620 patients undergoing coronary angioplasty. Arch Intern Med 2002;162:329–36.

44. Katholi RE, Woods WT Jr, Taylor GJ, et al. Oxygen free radicals and contrast nephropathy. Am J Kidney Dis 1998;32:64–71.

45. Merten GJ, Burgess WP, Gray LV, et al. Prevention of contrast-induced nephropathy with sodium bicarbonate: a randomized controlled trial. JAMA 2004;291:2328–34.

46. Ozcan EE, Guneri S, Akdeniz B, et al. Sodium bicarbonate, N-acetylcysteine, and saline for prevention of radiocontrast-induced nephropathy. A comparison of 3 regimens for protecting contrast-induced nephropathy in patients undergoing coronary procedures. A single-center prospective controlled trial. Am Heart J 2007;154:539–44.

47. Hoste EA, De Waele JJ, Gevaert SA, et al. Sodium bicarbonate for prevention of contrast-induced acute kidney injury: a systematic review and meta-analysis. Nephrol Dial Transplant 2010;25: 747–58.

48. Tepel M, van der Giet M, Schwarzfeld C, et al. Prevention of radiographic-contrast-agent-induced reductions in renal function by acetylcysteine. N Engl J Med 2000;343:180–4.

49. Recio-Mayoral A, Chaparro M, Prado B, et al. The reno-protective effect of hydration with sodium bicarbonate plus N-acetylcysteine in patients undergoing emergency percutaneous coronary intervention: the RENO Study. J Am Coll Cardiol 2007;49:1283–8.

50. Briguori C, Airoldi F, D'Andrea D, et al. Renal Insufficiency Following Contrast Media Administration Trial (REMEDIAL): a randomized comparison of 3 preventive strategies. Circulation 2007;115: 1211–7.

51. ACT Investigators. Acetylcysteine for prevention of renal outcomes in patients undergoing coronary and peripheral vascular angiography: main results from the randomized Acetylcysteine for Contrast-induced nephropathy Trial (ACT). Circulation 2011;124:1250–9.

52. Gurm HS, Smith DE, Berwanger O, et al. Contemporary use and effectiveness of N-acetylcysteine in preventing contrast-induced nephropathy among patients undergoing percutaneous coronary intervention. JACC Cardiovasc Interv 2012;5: 98–104.

53. Khanal S, Attallah N, Smith DE, et al. Statin therapy reduces contrast-induced nephropathy: an analysis of contemporary percutaneous interventions. Am J Med 2005;118:843–9.

54. Xinwei J, Xianghua F, Jing Z, et al. Comparison of usefulness of simvastatin 20 mg versus 80 mg in preventing contrast-induced nephropathy in patients with acute coronary syndrome undergoing percutaneous coronary intervention. Am J Cardiol 2009;104:519–24.

55. Patti G, Ricottini E, Nusca A, et al. Short-term, high-dose atorvastatin pretreatment to prevent contrast-induced nephropathy in patients with acute coronary syndromes undergoing percutaneous coronary intervention (from the ARMYDA-CIN [atorvastatin for reduction of myocardial damage during angioplasty–contrast-induced nephropathy] trial). Am J Cardiol 2011;108:1–7.

56. Quintavalle C, Fiore D, De Micco F, et al. Impact of a high loading dose of atorvastatin on contrast-induced acute kidney injury. Circulation 2012;126:3008–16.

57. Leoncini M, Toso A, Maioli M, et al. Early high-dose rosuvastatin for contrast-induced nephropathy prevention in acute coronary syndrome. Results from Protective effect of Rosuvastatin and Antiplatelet Therapy On contrast-induced acute kidney injury and myocardial damage in patients with Acute Coronary Syndrome (PRATO-ACS Study). J Am Coll Cardiol 2014;63(1):71–9.

58. Misbin RI, Green L, Stadel BV, et al. Lactic acidosis in patients with diabetes treated with metformin. N Engl J Med 1998;338:265–6.

59. Khurana R, Malik IS. Metformin: safety in cardiac patients. Heart 2010;96:99–102.

60. Maznyczka A, Myat A, Gershlick A. Discontinuation of metformin in the setting of coronary angiography: clinical uncertainty amongst physicians reflecting a poor evidence base. EuroIntervention 2012;7:1103–10.

61. Authors/Task Force Members, Ryden L, Grant PJ, et al. ESC Guidelines on diabetes, pre-diabetes, and cardiovascular diseases developed in collaboration with the EASD: the Task Force on diabetes, pre-diabetes, and cardiovascular diseases of the European Society of Cardiology (ESC) and developed in collaboration with the European Association for the Study of Diabetes (EASD). Eur Heart J 2013;34:3035–87.

62. Cirit M, Toprak O, Yesil M, et al. Angiotensin-converting enzyme inhibitors as a risk factor for contrast-induced nephropathy. Nephron Clin Pract 2006;104:c20–7.

63. Umruddin Z, Moe K, Superdock K. ACE inhibitor or angiotensin II receptor blocker use is a risk factor for contrast-induced nephropathy. J Nephrol 2012;25:776–81.

64. Gupta RK, Kapoor A, Tewari S, et al. Captopril for prevention of contrast-induced nephropathy in

diabetic patients: a randomised study. Indian Heart J 1999;51:521–6.

65. Rosenstock JL, Bruno R, Kim JK, et al. The effect of withdrawal of ACE inhibitors or angiotensin receptor blockers prior to coronary angiography on the incidence of contrast-induced nephropathy. Int Urol Nephrol 2008;40:749–55.

66. Cruz DN, Goh CY, Marenzi G, et al. Renal replacement therapies for prevention of radiocontrast-induced nephropathy: a systematic review. Am J Med 2012;125:66–78.e3.

67. Bader BD, Berger ED, Heede MB, et al. What is the best hydration regimen to prevent contrast media-induced nephrotoxicity? Clin Nephrol 2004;62:1–7.

68. Krasuski RA, Beard BM, Geoghagan JD, et al. Optimal timing of hydration to erase contrast-associated nephropathy: the OTHER CAN study. J Invasive Cardiol 2003;15:699–702.

69. Torigoe K, Tamura A, Watanabe T, et al. 20-Hour preprocedural hydration is not superior to 5-hour preprocedural hydration in the prevention of contrast-induced increases in serum creatinine and cystatin C. Int J Cardiol 2013;167:2200–3.

70. Stacul F, Adam A, Becker CR, et al. Strategies to reduce the risk of contrast-induced nephropathy. Am J Cardiol 2006;98:59K–77K.

71. Brar S. A prospective, randomized trial of sliding-scale hydration for prevention of contrast nephropathy; The POSEIDON (Prevention of Contrast Renal Injury with Different Hydration Strategies) trial. The Transcatheter Cardiovascular Therapeutics (TCT) conference. Miami, October 22-26, 2012.

72. Nayak KR, Mehta HS, Price MJ, et al. A novel technique for ultra-low contrast administration during angiography or intervention. Catheter Cardiovasc Interv 2010;75:1076–83.

Renal Complications in Patients Undergoing Peripheral Artery Interventions

Sachin S. Goel, MD[a], Mehdi H. Shishehbor, DO, MPH, PhD[b],*

KEYWORDS

- Contrast-induced nephropathy • Peripheral artery intervention • Calculated creatinine clearance
- Acute kidney injury

KEY POINTS

- Contrast-induced nephropathy (CIN) is the most important and most frequent renal complication of endovascular interventional procedures.
- The risk factors for CIN in this population are poorly defined. Small studies suggest that chronic kidney disease, diabetes, age older than 75 years, anemia, and volume of contrast used are risk factors for CIN.
- A ratio of contrast volume/calculated creatinine clearance (CV/CCC) that exceeds 3 is associated with significantly increased risk of CIN.
- Minimizing contrast use and adequate preprocedure and postprocedure hydration remains the main preventive strategy for CIN.

Peripheral artery disease (PAD) is a significant problem with increasing incidence and prevalence, particularly in the elderly.[1] The reported prevalence of PAD among individuals older than 70 years is 14.5%, which equals nearly 4 million adults in the United States.[2] The management of patients with severe PAD initially includes appropriate medical therapy and lifestyle changes for prevention of death, stroke, or myocardial infarction, in addition to symptom relief and prevention of amputation. Surgical or endovascular revascularization procedures are typically performed in patients with lifestyle-limiting symptoms or evidence of end-organ ischemia secondary to PAD.[3] The role of endovascular therapy in the treatment of PAD is expanding. Knowledge about complications and their prevention and management is essential for successful outcomes. This article focuses on renal complications during peripheral artery interventions.

CONTRAST-INDUCED NEPHROPATHY

Contrast-induced nephropathy (CIN) is the most important and most frequent renal complication of endovascular interventional procedures. A definition of CIN is given in **Box 1**.

Incidence

CIN is the third leading cause of acute kidney injury (AKI) in hospitalized patients, and is associated with significant patient morbidity.[7,8] It remains a common problem after coronary and peripheral arterial procedures, and occurs in 1% to 5% of low-risk patients; however, the incidence can be as high as 30% to 50% in high-risk populations.[9,10] In a report from the BMC2 PVI (Blue Cross Blue Shield of Michigan Cardiovascular Consortium Peripheral Vascular Intervention) Program, a prospective multicenter observational registry, of 7769 patients undergoing lower extremity

The authors have nothing to disclose.
[a] Interventional Cardiology, Department of Cardiovascular Medicine, Heart & Vascular Institute, 9500 Euclid Avenue, Cleveland, OH 44195, USA; [b] Endovascular Services, Heart & Vascular Institute, Cleveland Clinic, 9500 Euclid Avenue, Cleveland, OH 44195, USA
* Corresponding author.
E-mail address: shishem@ccf.org

interventional.theclinics.com

peripheral vascular interventions (LE PVI), the incidence of CIN was about 3% in patients younger than 70 years and 7% in those 80 years and older.[11]

Impact of CIN

Most data on CIN are derived from patients undergoing percutaneous coronary intervention (PCI); the predictors and implications of CIN in patients undergoing endovascular peripheral arterial interventions are poorly defined. However, patients undergoing peripheral arterial interventions often have coexistent atherosclerosis in the coronary and cerebral circulation, and have comorbidities similar to those in patients with coronary disease undergoing PCI. The incidence of CIN requiring dialysis is 0.3% in low-risk populations and as high as 12% to 15% in high-risk populations.[12] Multiple studies have shown the association between CIN and the increased risk of early and long-term adverse events such as myocardial infarction, rehospitalization, and mortality.[8,13] In a study from the Mayo Clinic assessing 7586 patients undergoing coronary interventions, the incidence of CIN was 3.3%, with a 22% in-hospital mortality rate in those who developed this complication.[8] Among survivors of CIN, the long-term rates of myocardial infarction and death were significantly higher in comparison with those without CIN. It is unclear, however, whether CIN is associated with a similar adverse hazard in patients undergoing peripheral interventions.

Pathophysiology

The exact underlying mechanism of CIN is unclear. The 2 main pathophysiologic mechanisms proposed include renal vasoconstriction with medullary hypoxia, leading to acute tubular necrosis (ATN) and direct cytotoxic effects of contrast agents.[14] Renal vasoconstriction is thought to be mediated by changes in the viscosity of blood to the medullary regions of the kidney by the contrast media, and partly by vasoactive mediators such as adenosine, nitric oxide, and endothelin.[15,16] Direct cytotoxic effects of contrast and generation of oxygen free radicals also contributes to the development of CIN.[14,17]

Risk Factors for CIN

Several patient-related and procedural factors have been recognized as risk factors for the development of CIN in patients undergoing PCI (Box 2). Risk models have been derived to predict the risk of CIN and to define safe limits of contrast media in patients undergoing PCI.[9,10] These risk models are heavily weighted by cardiogenic shock and hypotension, conditions that are infrequent among patients undergoing peripheral arterial procedures. Patients undergoing peripheral artery interventions, however, share other comorbidities with patients undergoing PCI, such as hypertension, diabetes mellitus, chronic kidney disease, congestive heart failure, and older age. Pending data from PAD-specific interventional procedures, these models developed in PCI patients should not be used in patients undergoing peripheral interventional procedures for risk assessment. Patient risk profiles are nonmodifiable to a large extent during the interventional procedure. Hence, studies have focused on identification of a safe upper limit of contrast volume that can be administered during procedures. In a large study from the BMC2 registry from 2007 to 2008, consisting of 58,957 patients undergoing PCI, the risk of CIN and nephropathy requiring dialysis (NRD) was found to be markedly increased when the ratio of contrast volume/calculated creatinine clearance (CV/CCC) exceeded 3 (odds ratio [OR] for CIN 1.46, 95% confidence interval [CI] 1.27–1.66; OR for NRD 1.89, 95% CI 1.24–2.94).[9] The CV/CCC ratio is a simple tool that helps minimize contrast dose in patients undergoing interventional procedures.

Clinical Course

CIN usually manifests only with an elevation in creatinine. The elevation in creatinine usually occurs 24 to 48 hours after contrast exposure, peaks at 3 to 5 days, and normalizes over 7 to 10 days after exposure. Most patients retain a normal urine output. In some patients, particularly those with baseline renal dysfunction, renal function will not recover completely, and some patients will progress to end-stage renal disease requiring dialysis.

Diagnosis

The diagnosis is usually based on the clinical presentation, including increase in creatinine 24 to 48 hours after contrast exposure and exclusion of other causes of AKI. Urinalysis may show muddy brown casts and epithelial cell casts on urine sedimentation suggestive of ATN, the pathophysiologic hallmark of CIN. Presence of white cell casts, red cell casts, or eosinophils suggests alternative diagnoses such as interstitial nephritis, glomerular disease, or renal atheroembolism, respectively, which are in the differential diagnosis of CIN. Renal atheroembolism is discussed in some more detail later in this article. Renal ultrasonography is usually not necessary in patients with a classic presentation and course suggestive of CIN, but can be useful in excluding other causes of AKI if suspected.

CONTRAST AGENTS

Contrast media are discussed in greater detail in several other articles in this issue by Buschur and colleagues; only factors relevant to peripheral interventions are reviewed here. Contrast agents are benzoic acid derivatives with 3 iodine atoms replacing the hydrogen atoms at positions 2, 4, and 6 of the benzene ring. These agents are classified based on charge of the iodinated molecule (ionic vs nonionic), molecular structure (monomeric or dimeric), and osmolality (hyperosmolal, low-osmolal, or iso-osmolal, relative to normal serum osmolality of 270–290 mOsm/kg).

The characteristics of contrast agents responsible for nephrotoxicity are not known, although both osmolality and viscosity have been implicated. In general, high-osmolar agents are not used in peripheral arterial interventions because of the significant side effects and pain. Almost all such procedures are performed with iso-osmolar or certain select low-osmolar contrast media. Some studies have suggested that an iso-osmolar nonionic dimer, iodixanol (osmolality = 290 mOsm/kg) was associated with a lower risk of CIN in comparison with low-osmolar agents.[18,19] Data from recent meta-analyses of randomized trials suggest that there is no significant difference in the risk of CIN with the use of iodixanol compared with a pool of ionic and nonionic low-osmolar contrast media (LOCM).[20,21] Stratified analyses showed that iodixanol was associated with a relatively lower rate of CIN when compared with ioxaglate (low-osmolar ionic dimer) or iohexol (low-osmolar nonionic agent), but there was no difference in CIN when comparing iodixanol with other low-osmolar nonionic agents such as iopromide and iopamidol.[20] In patients with baseline renal dysfunction, iodixanol was found to be associated with reduced risk of CIN compared with iohexol, but not other LOCM.[21]

In general, the choice of contrast media for peripheral arterial procedures is dictated by patient discomfort associated with agents that have higher osmolality, and it is unclear as to whether the contrast agents used for contemporary endovascular procedures impart a different risk of CIN.

PREVENTION AND MANAGEMENT OF CIN

There is no specific treatment for CIN, and management is similar to that for other causes of ATN, such as maintaining fluid and electrolyte balance and avoiding further nephrotoxins including repeated contrast exposure. The best treatment is prevention. The first step in preventing CIN is assessment of individual patient risk factors (see earlier discussion) before performing the diagnostic or interventional procedure. Even though serum creatinine has been used to assess baseline renal function, it has limitations. Calculating the creatinine clearance using the Cockcroft-Gault formula or the estimated glomerular filtration rate (eGFR) using the MDRD (Modification of Diet in Renal Disease) equation is a more accurate way of assessing baseline renal function. Several strategies have been studied for the prevention of CIN; however, the 2 consistently proven ones are hydration and limiting contrast volume.

Hydration

Adequate preprocedure and postprocedure hydration remains the main preventive strategy for CIN. This subject is extensively reviewed in "Intravenous and Oral Hydration: Approaches, Principals and Differing Regimens" by Igor Rojkovskiy and Richard Solomon elsewhere in this issue. It has been shown that volume expansion with isotonic saline is superior to one-half isotonic saline.[22] Prolonged hydration, namely 6 to 12 hours before and 12 to 24 hours after the procedure, is preferable to bolus administration. Urinary alkalization with sodium bicarbonate may protect against CIN via an effect on reactive oxygen species. The results of studies evaluating this strategy have been conflicting, with some studies showing reduced incidence of CIN with sodium bicarbonate[23–25] and others demonstrating no benefit.[26–28] At present the data are inconclusive in support of one of either saline-based or sodium bicarbonate–based hydration strategy over the other. The authors recommend that each institution should have a standardized protocol to hydrate patients who are presumed to be at high risk for CIN. At the authors' center, this includes patients with an eGFR of less than 60 mL/min/1.73 m^2.

Pharmacologic-Based and Device-Based Prevention

Different drug-based and device-based approaches have been or are being studied for the prevention of CIN, mainly in patients undergoing PCI. The outcomes of these studies will certainly apply to patients undergoing peripheral artery interventions. At present there are no specific drugs or devices that have been approved for use in patients undergoing peripheral arterial procedures.

Limiting Contrast Volume

The volume of contrast used must always be considered during a procedure in light of baseline renal function and other risk factors present in the individual patient. Several studies have evaluated "safe levels" of contrast. Studies have used and validated maximal acceptable contrast dose, which is calculated by 5 mL of contrast × body weight (kg)/baseline serum creatinine (mg/dL).[29] Subsequently, the CV/CCC ratio was evaluated in 3179 patients undergoing coronary intervention, and a ratio higher than 3.7 was found to be associated with significantly increased risk of CIN.[30] As mentioned earlier, a large study from the BMC2 registry consisting of 58,957 patients demonstrated that the risk of CIN was found to be markedly increased when the CV/CCC ratio exceeded 3.[9] The CV/CCC ratio is a simple tool that helps minimize contrast dose in patients undergoing interventional procedures.

In patients undergoing peripheral arterial interventions, many techniques can be used to minimize contrast volume, including ultralow volume contrast technique during angiography and/or intervention as described by Nayak and colleagues.[31] The key elements of this approach include the use of no more than 1 to 2 cm^3 of contrast per injection, which is achieved by mixing saline with contrast in a ratio of 70:30 or 80:20; biplane angiography; use of intravascular ultrasonography (IVUS) to determine lesion length, lesion severity, vessel diameter, and balloon and stent size; removing contrast from the guide catheter or sheath by back bleeding or aspirating before exchange of devices; use of the road-map technique while crossing lesions; balloon and stent placement; using prior angiographic images, if available, as a reference for guidance during guide wire, balloon, and stent passage; and staging diagnostic and interventional procedures, when required, by at least 72 hours.

Carbon dioxide (CO_2) angiography is another technique that has been used in patients allergic to iodinated contrast media and those at high risk for CIN.[32] In addition to being nonallergic and nonnephrotoxic, the advantages of CO_2 include its low viscosity and central reflux, allowing accurate assessment of proximal vessels on injection without withdrawing the catheter. Disadvantages include invisibility with potential for air contamination, need for a special delivery system, potential hypotension and bradycardia with injection of excessive volumes of CO_2, and contraindication for use in coronary and cerebral circulation. It is generally believed that CO_2 angiography is safer than contrast angiography, and there is no reported case of AKI when CO_2 angiography has been used for lower extremity procedures. Even among patients undergoing abdominal aortic or renal procedures, CO_2 has been generally safe; however, there are rare case reports of bowel and renal ischemia following CO_2 angiography, although in such cases air or cholesterol embolization could not be excluded.[33]

In the past gadolinium was used as an alternative contrast agent. However, after reports linking use of gadolinium and occurrence of nephrogenic systemic fibrosis emerged in 2006, its use has practically been discontinued in those with or at risk of renal dysfunction, in accordance with current guidelines.[34]

COMPLICATIONS DURING RENAL ARTERY INTERVENTION

Renal artery stenosis has been implicated in resistant hypertension, chronic kidney disease, and flash or recurrent pulmonary edema. Renal artery stenting has been a prevalent procedure, despite its controversial role. Worsening of renal function is a well-known complication of this procedure. CIN is always a potential risk in endovascular procedures (see discussion in the preceding section). Renal atheroembolization is a major concern in this population, and all steps must be taken to minimize it. In the authors' experience IVUS is a valuable tool for guiding renal artery stenting, particularly in those with baseline renal dysfunction. IVUS is able to characterize the lesion, assess lesion length and vessel size, determine the location of the ostium of the renal artery for precise stent placement, and evaluate the vessel for complications and need for postdilatation, thus reducing the use of contrast and decreasing the risk of CIN during renal artery stenting.

Atheroembolization

Atheroembolization can occur during renal artery stenting and can manifest with renal failure. It can be accompanied by nonspecific symptoms such as fever, myalgia, weight loss, headaches, or embolization to other organs, particularly skin of toes and feet, with evidence of blue toes or livedo reticularis. Presence of extensive and diffuse atherosclerosis in the abdominal aorta and renal arteries increases the risk of this complication. Manipulation of catheters in the abdominal aorta, or engaging the ostium of the renal artery during angiography and intervention can lead to disruption of plaque followed by embolization. There is no specific treatment for this condition. Management is largely supportive and includes consideration given to withdrawal of anticoagulation, avoidance of repeated contrast exposure, analgesia, foot care, and dialysis. Renal atheroembolism is associated with poor prognosis. In a study consisting of 354 patients with renal atheroembolism followed for 2 years (271 patients had iatrogenic cause after angiography or intervention), 33% of patients required dialysis within 6 months of the event, and mortality was 25% at 2 years.[35] Hence prevention is the most important strategy. Careful manipulation of catheters in the abdominal aorta, use of 5F soft-tipped catheters for diagnostic angiography, use of the no-touch technique, use of IVUS, careful bleeding back to clear the system of blood and potential debris, and flushing before injection may reduce the risk of this complication. The no-touch technique involves placing a 0.035-in (0.889-mm) guide wire in the guide catheter beyond the tip during cannulation of the renal artery with a steerable guide wire (the authors prefer a 0.018-in [0.457-mm] guide wire) to prevent the tip of the guide catheter from rubbing against the aortic wall, thus minimizing the risk of disruption of atherosclerotic plaque and embolization.[36]

Renal Artery Dissection

Renal artery dissection can result from aggressive manipulation of the catheter during engagement or disengagement of the ostium, or balloon or stent oversizing. Single-center studies have reported a 1% to 3% rate of renal artery dissection after renal artery stenting.[37,38] If the dissection is flow limiting or there is a significant pressure gradient across the dissected segment, it can be treated by an endovascular technique using prolonged balloon inflation to tack the dissection flap, or stenting if the balloon angioplasty is unsuccessful.

Renal Artery Perforation

Distal renal artery perforation from a guide wire is an uncommon but potentially fatal complication.[39,40] The incidence has been reported to be 1% or less. Symptoms can include ipsilateral flank pain, hypotension, and shock. Prompt recognition during angiography is important for timely management. Therapy includes reversal of anticoagulation, arterial occlusion with a balloon, coil embolization, and/or covered stent placement. Renal artery rupture can occur as a result of oversizing of the balloon or stent.[37,41] Management includes reversal of anticoagulation, covered stent placement, and surgical repair.

Renal Artery Thrombosis and Occlusion

Renal artery thrombosis and occlusion can occur as a result of flow-limiting dissection, inadequate anticoagulation during intervention, underlying hypercoagulable state, and heparin-induced thrombocytopenia. The incidence is less than 1%.[42] Therapy includes adequate anticoagulation and treatment of underlying abnormality.

Renal Infarction

The incidence of renal infarction ranges from 1% to 2%.[37] Underlying causes include atheroembolism, renal artery perforation, thrombosis, and flow-limiting dissection. Clinical manifestations include severe flank pain, hematuria, and nausea. Diagnosis is confirmed by computed tomography or angiography. Management includes analgesia, hydration, reversal of anticoagulation, and endovascular management in cases of perforation.

RENAL COMPLICATIONS DURING ENDOVASCULAR AORTIC INTERVENTIONS

Endovascular aneurysm repair (EVAR) has been an important advance in the management of abdominal aortic aneurysm (AAA). Studies comparing open AAA repair with EVAR have shown improved short-term morbidity and mortality with EVAR, but no significant difference in long-term outcomes.[43,44] As a result, there has been a significant increase in the number of EVARs being performed in the United States, likely a result of patients who would not have been candidates for open AAA repair now being candidates for EVAR. Intravenous contrast is used during EVAR to assist in proper graft positioning. Consequently, CIN remains a risk after EVAR. In a retrospective study involving more than 6500 patients undergoing EVAR, the incidence of AKI was 6.7%.[45] The incidence of renal failure requiring dialysis after EVAR is in the range of 0.8% to 2%.[45,46] Renal ischemia can be caused during EVAR by renal artery embolism, thrombosis, dissection, or impingement of the origin of the renal artery by the endograft.[47] The latter complication can occur with endograft placement in the setting of a short aortic neck. Repositioning the graft, stenting the occluded renal artery, or surgical bypass are the treatment options once renal artery coverage occurs. Suprarenal fixation devices have been used with EVAR; however, the effect of this technique in the prevention of renal dysfunction following EVAR is debatable.[48]

REFERENCES

1. Norgren L, Hiatt WR, Dormandy JA, et al. Inter-society consensus for the management of peripheral arterial disease (TASC II). J Vasc Surg 2007; 45(Suppl S):S5–67.

2. Selvin E, Erlinger TP. Prevalence of and risk factors for peripheral arterial disease in the United States: results from the National Health and Nutrition Examination Survey, 1999-2000. Circulation 2004;110: 738–43.

3. Hirsch AT, Haskal ZJ, Hertzer NR, et al. ACC/AHA 2005 guidelines for the management of patients with peripheral arterial disease (lower extremity, renal, mesenteric, and abdominal aortic): executive summary a collaborative report from the American Association for Vascular Surgery/Society for Vascular Surgery, Society for Cardiovascular Angiography and Interventions, Society for Vascular Medicine and Biology, Society of Interventional Radiology, and the ACC/AHA Task Force on Practice Guidelines (Writing Committee to Develop Guidelines for the Management of Patients With Peripheral Arterial Disease) endorsed by the American Association of Cardiovascular and Pulmonary Rehabilitation; National Heart, Lung, and Blood Institute; Society for Vascular Nursing; TransAtlantic Inter-Society Consensus; and Vascular Disease Foundation. J Am Coll Cardiol 2006;47:1239–312.

4. Barrett BJ, Parfrey PS. Clinical practice. Preventing nephropathy induced by contrast medium. N Engl J Med 2006;354:379–86.

5. Murphy SW, Barrett BJ, Parfrey PS. Contrast nephropathy. J Am Soc Nephrol 2000;11:177–82.

6. Solomon R, Dauerman HL. Contrast-induced acute kidney injury. Circulation 2010;122:2451–5.

7. Nash K, Hafeez A, Hou S. Hospital-acquired renal insufficiency. Am J Kidney Dis 2002;39:930–6.

8. Rihal CS, Textor SC, Grill DE, et al. Incidence and prognostic importance of acute renal failure after percutaneous coronary intervention. Circulation 2002;105:2259–64.

9. Gurm HS, Dixon SR, Smith DE, et al. Renal function-based contrast dosing to define safe limits of radiographic contrast media in patients undergoing percutaneous coronary interventions. J Am Coll Cardiol 2011;58:907–14.

10. Mehran R, Aymong ED, Nikolsky E, et al. A simple risk score for prediction of contrast-induced nephropathy after percutaneous coronary intervention: development and initial validation. J Am Coll Cardiol 2004;44:1393–9.

11. Plaisance BR, Munir K, Share DA, et al. Safety of contemporary percutaneous peripheral arterial interventions in the elderly insights from the BMC2 PVI (Blue Cross Blue Shield of Michigan Cardiovascular Consortium Peripheral Vascular Intervention) registry. JACC Cardiovasc Interv 2011;4:694–701.

12. Kane GC, Doyle BJ, Lerman A, et al. Ultra-low contrast volumes reduce rates of contrast-induced nephropathy in patients with chronic kidney disease undergoing coronary angiography. J Am Coll Cardiol 2008;51:89–90.

13. James MT, Ghali WA, Knudtson ML, et al. Associations between acute kidney injury and cardiovascular and renal outcomes after coronary angiography. Circulation 2011;123:409–16.

14. Persson PB, Hansell P, Liss P. Pathophysiology of contrast medium-induced nephropathy. Kidney Int 2005;68:14–22.

15. Cantley LG, Spokes K, Clark B, et al. Role of endothelin and prostaglandins in radiocontrast-induced renal artery constriction. Kidney Int 1993;44: 1217–23.

16. Katholi RE, Taylor GJ, McCann WP, et al. Nephrotoxicity from contrast media: attenuation with theophylline. Radiology 1995;195:17–22.

17. Heinrich MC, Kuhlmann MK, Grgic A, et al. Cytotoxic effects of ionic high-osmolar, nonionic monomeric, and nonionic iso-osmolar dimeric iodinated contrast media on renal tubular cells in vitro. Radiology 2005; 235:843–9.

18. Aspelin P, Aubry P, Fransson SG, et al. Nephrotoxic effects in high-risk patients undergoing angiography. N Engl J Med 2003;348:491–9.

19. Jo SH, Youn TJ, Koo BK, et al. Renal toxicity evaluation and comparison between Visipaque (iodixanol) and Hexabrix (ioxaglate) in patients with renal insufficiency undergoing coronary angiography: the RECOVER study: a randomized controlled trial. J Am Coll Cardiol 2006;48:924–30.

20. Reed M, Meier P, Tamhane UU, et al. The relative renal safety of iodixanol compared with low-osmolar contrast media: a meta-analysis of randomized controlled trials. JACC Cardiovasc Interv 2009; 2:645–54.

21. Heinrich MC, Haberle L, Muller V, et al. Nephrotoxicity of iso-osmolar iodixanol compared with nonionic low-osmolar contrast media: meta-analysis of randomized controlled trials. Radiology 2009;250:68–86.

22. Mueller C, Buerkle G, Buettner HJ, et al. Prevention of contrast media-associated nephropathy: randomized comparison of 2 hydration regimens in 1620 patients undergoing coronary angioplasty. Arch Intern Med 2002;162:329–36.

23. Merten GJ, Burgess WP, Gray LV, et al. Prevention of contrast-induced nephropathy with sodium bicarbonate: a randomized controlled trial. JAMA 2004; 291:2328–34.

24. Briguori C, Airoldi F, D'Andrea D, et al. Renal Insufficiency Following Contrast Media Administration Trial (REMEDIAL): a randomized comparison of 3 preventive strategies. Circulation 2007;115:1211–7.

25. Recio-Mayoral A, Chaparro M, Prado B, et al. The reno-protective effect of hydration with sodium bicarbonate plus N-acetylcysteine in patients undergoing emergency percutaneous coronary intervention: the RENO Study. J Am Coll Cardiol 2007;49: 1283–8.

26. Brar SS, Shen AY, Jorgensen MB, et al. Sodium bicarbonate vs sodium chloride for the prevention of contrast medium-induced nephropathy in patients undergoing coronary angiography: a randomized trial. JAMA 2008;300:1038–46.

27. Maioli M, Toso A, Leoncini M, et al. Sodium bicarbonate versus saline for the prevention of contrast-induced nephropathy in patients with renal dysfunction undergoing coronary angiography or intervention. J Am Coll Cardiol 2008;52:599–604.

28. Vasheghani-Farahani A, Sadigh G, Kassaian SE, et al. Sodium bicarbonate plus isotonic saline versus saline for prevention of contrast-induced nephropathy in patients undergoing coronary angiography: a randomized controlled trial. Am J Kidney Dis 2009; 54:610–8.

29. Cigarroa RG, Lange RA, Williams RH, et al. Dosing of contrast material to prevent contrast nephropathy in patients with renal disease. Am J Med 1989;86: 649–52.

30. Laskey WK, Jenkins C, Selzer F, et al. Volume-to-creatinine clearance ratio: a pharmacokinetically based risk factor for prediction of early creatinine increase after percutaneous coronary intervention. J Am Coll Cardiol 2007;50:584–90.

31. Nayak KR, Mehta HS, Price MJ, et al. A novel technique for ultra-low contrast administration during angiography or intervention. Catheter Cardiovasc Interv 2010;75:1076–83.

32. Hawkins IF, Cho KJ, Caridi JG. Carbon dioxide in angiography to reduce the risk of contrast-induced nephropathy. Radiol Clin North Am 2009;47:813–25, v–vi.

33. Johnson PL, Neperud J, Arnold J, et al. Livedo reticularis and bowel ischemia after carbon dioxide arteriography in a patient with CREST syndrome. J Vasc Interv Radiol 2011;22:395–9.

34. Thomsen HS. How to avoid nephrogenic systemic fibrosis: current guidelines in Europe and the United States. Radiol Clin North Am 2009;47:871–5, vii.

35. Scolari F, Ravani P, Gaggi R, et al. The challenge of diagnosing atheroembolic renal disease: clinical features and prognostic factors. Circulation 2007; 116:298–304.

36. Feldman RL, Wargovich TJ, Bittl JA. No-touch technique for reducing aortic wall trauma during renal artery stenting. Catheter Cardiovasc Interv 1999;46: 245–8.

37. Ivanovic V, McKusick MA, Johnson CM 3rd, et al. Renal artery stent placement: complications at a single tertiary care center. J Vasc Interv Radiol 2003; 14:217–25.

38. Beek FJ, Kaatee R, Beutler JJ, et al. Complications during renal artery stent placement for atherosclerotic ostial stenosis. Cardiovasc Intervent Radiol 1997;20:184–90.

39. Axelrod DJ, Freeman H, Pukin L, et al. Guide wire perforation leading to fatal perirenal hemorrhage from transcortical collaterals after renal artery stent placement. J Vasc Interv Radiol 2004;15:985–7.

40. Heye S, Vanbeckevoort D, Blockmans D, et al. Iatrogenic main renal artery injury: treatment by endovascular stent-graft placement. Cardiovasc Intervent Radiol 2005;28:93–4.

41. Oguzkurt L, Tercan F, Gulcan O, et al. Rupture of the renal artery after cutting balloon angioplasty in a young woman with fibromuscular dysplasia. Cardiovasc Intervent Radiol 2005;28:360–3.

42. Bush RL, Najibi S, MacDonald MJ, et al. Endovascular revascularization of renal artery stenosis: technical and clinical results. J Vasc Surg 2001;33: 1041–9.

43. Greenhalgh RM, Brown LC, Powell JT, et al. Endovascular versus open repair of abdominal aortic aneurysm. N Engl J Med 2010;362:1863–71.

44. De Bruin JL, Baas AF, Buth J, et al. Long-term outcome of open or endovascular repair of abdominal aortic aneurysm. N Engl J Med 2010;362:1881–9.

45. Wald R, Waikar SS, Liangos O, et al. Acute renal failure after endovascular vs open repair of abdominal aortic aneurysm. J Vasc Surg 2006;43:460–6 [discussion: 466].

46. Lederle FA, Freischlag JA, Kyriakides TC, et al. Outcomes following endovascular vs open repair of abdominal aortic aneurysm: a randomized trial. JAMA 2009;302:1535–42.

47. Brown LC, Brown EA, Greenhalgh RM, et al. Renal function and abdominal aortic aneurysm (AAA): the impact of different management strategies on long-term renal function in the UK EndoVascular Aneurysm Repair (EVAR) Trials. Ann Surg 2010;251:966–75.

48. Greenberg RK, Chuter TA, Lawrence-Brown M, et al. Analysis of renal function after aneurysm repair with a device using suprarenal fixation (Zenith AAA Endovascular Graft) in contrast to open surgical repair. J Vasc Surg 2004;39:1219–28.

Renal Complications in Patients Undergoing Transcatheter Aortic Valve Replacement

Justin M. Dunn, MD, MPH[a], E. Murat Tuzcu, MD[a],
Samir R. Kapadia, MD[b],*

KEYWORDS

- Renal insufficiency • TAVR • Acute kidney injury • Kidney

KEY POINTS

- Chronic kidney disease increases the risk of transcatheter aortic valve replacement (TAVR) in the high-risk symptomatic patients that are typically referred for this procedure.
- In preprocedural planning, minimizing contrast dose is critical for preventing further renal compromise before TAVR.
- Biplane angiography, computed tomography with intra-arterial contrast injection, use of three-dimensional TEE, or cardiac magnetic resonance imaging for annular measurement and proper hydration before contrast administration can help to ameliorate the risk of acute kidney injury (AKI) following TAVR.
- Minimizing contrast during the procedure and preventing hemodynamic perturbations in the operative and perioperative period are of paramount importance in decreasing the risk of AKI following TAVR.
- Ultimate success of TAVR depends on careful attention to detail and expeditious management of complications.

INTRODUCTION

Acute kidney injury (AKI) in hospitalized patients is associated with significantly increased mortality across a broad spectrum of conditions.[1] According to the Society of Thoracic Surgeons database, patients with chronic kidney disease (CKD) undergoing surgical aortic valve replacement (SAVR) with or without coronary artery bypass grafting had a more than 50% reduction in observed 8-year survival compared with those without CKD.[2] Depending on the definition used, the incidence of AKI following SAVR approaches 25% in some studies.[3] Transcatheter aortic valve replacement (TAVR) is an exciting new approach for the treatment of aortic stenosis in high-risk[4] or inoperable[5] patients with severe aortic stenosis.[6] This article discusses the incidence, predictors, impact, and potential avoidance and management strategies of renal dysfunction associated with TAVR.

INCIDENCE

The initial reports of AKI after TAVR varied widely based on a lack of standardized definitions. In the PARTNER trial, AKI was considered to be a creatinine level greater than 3 mg/dL or the need for new renal-replacement therapy after randomization. In cohort A (TAVR vs SAVR) and cohort B (TAVR vs medical therapy ± balloon valvuloplasty)

The authors have nothing to disclose.
[a] Cleveland Clinic, 9500 Euclid Avenue, J2-3, Cleveland, OH 44195, USA; [b] Cardiac Catheterization Laboratory, Cleveland Clinic, 9500 Euclid Avenue, J2-3, Cleveland, OH 44195, USA
* Corresponding author.
E-mail address: KAPADIS@ccf.org

Intervent Cardiol Clin 3 (2014) 449–454
http://dx.doi.org/10.1016/j.iccl.2014.03.003

there was no difference in the incidence of AKI between the groups at 30 days or at 1 year. In cohort A the incidence at 30 days was 4.1% and 4.2% in the TAVR and SAVR groups, respectively, and at 1 year was 9.3% and 9.2%, respectively.

In 2011, the Valve Academic Research Consortium (VARC) published standardized end point definitions for transcatheter aortic valve implantation clinical trials to improve clinical research quality and comparison among studies.[7] They initially suggested adopting serum creatinine criteria from the "modified" RIFLE (Risk, Injury, Failure, Loss, End-Stage kidney disease) classification (**Box 1**).[7] Using this definition, the incidence of significant AKI (stage 2–3) in 218 consecutive PARTNER trial patients at one institution from 2008 to 2011 was 8.3%.[8] Of note, the incidence of stage 1 AKI in this study was 26.1%. Other studies using the original VARC definitions report an incidence of stage 2 to 3 AKI ranging from 1.4% to 35.9%, with a pooled estimate rate of 8.0% to 8.4%.[9]

In 2012, however, the VARC released updated definitions[10] and their recommended definition changed to using the Acute Kidney Injury Network classification,[11] which is a modified version of the RIFLE classification that has been adopted by many in the nephrology community (**Box 2**). Using

---

Box 1
Acute kidney injury (modified RIFLE classification): original VARC definition

Change in serum creatinine (up to 72 hours) compared with baseline

- Stage 1: Increase in serum creatinine to 150%–200% (1.5–2.0× increase compared with baseline) OR increase of >0.3 mg/dL (>26.4 mmol/L)
- Stage 2: Increase in serum creatinine to 200%–300% (2.0–3.0× increase compared with baseline) OR increase between >0.3 mg/dL (>26.4 mmol/L) and <4.0 mg/dL (<354 mmol/L)
- Stage 3[a]: Increase in serum creatinine to ≥300% (>3× increase compared with baseline) OR serum creatinine of ≥4.0 mg/dL (≥354 mmol/L) with an acute increase of at least 0.5 mg/dL (44 mmol/L)

[a] Patients receiving renal replacement therapy are considered to meet Stage 3 criteria irrespective of other criteria.
From Leon MB, Piazza N, Nikolsky E, et al. Standardized endpoint definitions for transcatheter aortic valve implantation clinical trials: a consensus report from the Valve Academic Research Consortium. J Am Coll Cardiol 2011;57(3):258; with permission.

Box 2
Acute kidney injury (AKIN classification): updated VARC 2 definition

Stage 1

Increase in serum creatinine to 150%–199% (1.5–1.99× increase compared with baseline) OR

Increase of ≥0.3 mg/dL (≥26.4 mmol/L) OR

Urine output <0.5 mL/kg/h for >6 but <12 hours

Stage 2

Increase in serum creatinine to 200%–299% (2.0–2.99× increase compared with baseline) OR

Urine output <0.5 mL/kg/h for >12 but <24 hours

Stage 3[a]

Increase in serum creatinine to ≥300% (>3× increase compared with baseline) OR

Serum creatinine of ≥4.0 mg/dL (≥354 mmol/L) with an acute increase of at least 0.5 mg/dL (44 mmol/L) OR

Urine output <0.3 mL/kg/h for ≥24 hours OR

Anuria for ≥12 hours

The increase in creatinine must occur within 48 hours.
[a] Patients receiving renal replacement therapy are considered to meet Stage 3 criteria irrespective of other criteria.
From Kappetein AP, Head SJ, Genereax P, et al. Updated standardized endpoint definitions for transcatheter aortic valve implantation: the Valve Academic Research Consortium-2 consensus document. J Thorac Cardiovasc Surg 2012;145(1):13; with permission.

---

this new definition, the incidence of significant AKI (stage 2–3) in one study of 251 consecutive patients undergoing TAVR was 1.6%.[12] Of note, in this study the incidence of stage 1 AKI was 15.1% and of stage 3 AKI was 0% with no patients requiring renal-replacement therapy.

PREDICTORS

Several potential risk factors have been proposed as independent predictors of AKI following TAVR. The most common and consistent risk factors based on current data are discussed next.

Pre-existing Renal Dysfunction

In one study of 234 patients who underwent TAVR between 2007 and 2010 at a single center, pre-TAVR creatinine was the only independent predictor of AKI using multivariable logistic regression analysis.[13] There is also some suggestion that a higher CKD stage predicts AKI after TAVR.[14] However, most studies have failed to identify pre-existing renal dysfunction as an independent predictor of AKI post-TAVR.[15–20] In some of these studies creatinine actually improved after TAVR, likely because of reversal of some of the pathophysiologic consequences of the cardiorenal syndrome.

Peripheral Vascular Disease

Patients with significant vascular disease generally have a higher atherosclerotic burden, increasing the risk of atheroembolic disease during TAVR. In some studies, peripheral vascular disease was found to be an independent predictor of AKI following TAVR.[14,21] In these studies, however, the type and severity of peripheral vascular disease are not clearly defined.

Transapical Approach

Several studies have found the transapical approach to be an independent predictor of AKI after TAVR.[15,18,19] The mechanisms behind why the transapical approach would cause more AKI than the transfemoral approach are only speculative, but the most likely explanation is that patients who undergo transapical TAVR have more advanced vascular disease, which as discussed is a risk factor for AKI after TAVR.

Periprocedural Bleeding and Blood Transfusion

Several studies have identified periprocedural blood transfusion as an independent risk factor for AKI after TAVR.[18,20,21] Other studies have found life-threatening bleeding, defined according to VARC criteria, to be an independent risk factor.[8,22] One study found the number of periprocedural blood transfusions to be the strongest predictor of AKI following TAVR, but not the clinical indications for transfusion (ie, baseline anemia, vascular bleeding complications, blood loss).[21] This suggests that the transfusion itself is contributing to the AKI. The mechanism behind this is not well elucidated, but it has been shown that preserved red blood cells used in transfusions undergo structural changes during storage, such as reduced deformability and increased tendency to aggregate, which may contribute to their harmful effects.[23] Transfusions may also induce a systemic inflammatory response,[24] and in some studies an increased postprocedural leukocyte count is associated with AKI after TAVR.[20,21] Bleeding may induce hypotension and renal hypoperfusion.

Logistic EuroSCORE

The EuroSCORE is a risk model that includes several patient-related variables and is used to predict a patient's risk of death following cardiac surgery. Several studies have found a higher logistic EuroSCORE to be an independent predictor of AKI following TAVR.[20–22] It should be noted that "extracardiac arteriopathy," the definition that has significant overlap with the definition of peripheral vascular disease, is included in the logistic EuroSCORE.

Diabetes

The microvascular and macrovascular complications of diabetes may make the kidneys more susceptible to insults, such as hypotension and contrast administration. In one study the variable with the strongest independent association with the risk of AKI after TAVR was diabetes.[14] In another small study, diabetes and preprocedural renal dysfunction were the only two independent predictors of AKI following TAVR.[25]

Other Risk Factors

Some other possible predictors of AKI following TAVR in various studies include hypertension, previous myocardial infarction, chronic obstructive pulmonary disease, pulmonary hypertension, postprocedural aortic regurgitation, and postprocedural thrombocytopenia.

OUTCOMES
Mortality

AKI after TAVR is significantly associated with 30-day and 1-year mortality, and the risk of mortality increases with higher stage AKI.[14,26] The magnitude of the effect of AKI on mortality depends on the definition of AKI, but one study demonstrated that AKI is associated with a four-fold higher postoperative mortality following TAVR independent of baseline risk profile characteristics and periprocedural complications.[17]

Cost and Length of Stay in Hospital

Multiple studies have shown that AKI significantly increases the cost of care and length of stay in hospital across all conditions, including TAVR.[1,15,27,28]

AVOIDANCE AND MANAGEMENT STRATEGIES
Pigtail Computed Tomography

In patients without significant underlying renal insufficiency, the standard multidetector computed tomography protocol in patients planning for TAVR involves contrast injection through a peripheral intravenous (IV) line followed by gated high-resolution images of the aortic root and the heart, and nongated imaging of the entire ascending and descending aorta extending to the mid-thigh (**Fig. 1**).[29] In patients with impaired renal function, an alternative protocol has been described using a 4F pigtail catheter in the abdominal aorta. A computed tomography scan of the distal aorta and peripheral vessels is obtained using a mix of contrast and saline injected into the pigtail catheter at 4 mL/second for 10 seconds, using as little as 12 mL of contrast rather than the typical 80 to 150 mL of contrast typically used during the standard TAVR protocol multidetector computed tomography.

Transthoracic and Transesophageal Echocardiogram

Two- and three-dimensional transthoracic echocardiogram and transesophageal echocardiogram (TEE) are routinely used to evaluate the aortic valve and annulus before, during, and after TAVR.[30] Ultrasound imaging does not require the administration of contrast, which is an obvious advantage in patients with renal insufficiency. These imaging modalities, however, often underestimate the true aortic annulus and can be problematic in patients with heavy calcification of the aortic valve, which is common in the TAVR population.[31] There is some emerging evidence, however, that TEE

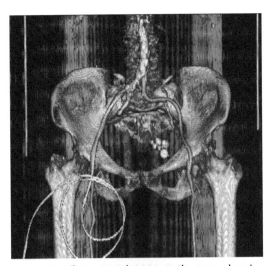

Fig. 1. Pigtail computed tomography scan showing the pelvic aorta and iliofemoral arterial system with a 4F pigtail catheter (seen coiled outside the body) inserted into the right common femoral artery by a 5F catheter sheath. The end of the pigtail catheter is resting just above the iliac bifurcation.

can be used as the primary imaging modality to guide TAVR procedures, especially transapical TAVR, possibly replacing the aortic root imaging performed with fluoroscopy and contrast administration.[32] Not all TAVR operators agree, however, and the role of TEE to minimize contrast administration is still being defined.[33]

Cardiac Magnetic Resonance

Cardiac magnetic resonance (CMR) allows for anatomic and functional assessment of the aortic valve and root without the need for IV contrast, providing an advantage in patients with baseline renal insufficiency. However, most CMR sequences are two-dimensional and the plane of the image often does not fully capture the complexity of the aortic annulus dimensions. In addition, calcium can cause signal void on CMR. Whole-heart, echo-gated, three-dimensional CMR with contrast can provide a better assessment of the shape and dimensions of the annulus. CMR is also becoming more useful in the assessment of patients post-TAVR, allowing for evaluation of valve integrity, position, aortic regurgitation, and postprocedure complications.[34]

Minimize Periprocedural Hypotension

As discussed, bleeding has been associated with increased AKI and worse outcomes following TAVR. This is likely caused by renal hypoperfusion secondary to hypotension and hypovolemia. Episodes of rapid pacing used during TAVR cause transient hypotension and pose a theoretical risk of AKI, but one study that evaluated the number of procedural pacing runs in the development of AKI following TAVR found no correlation.[17] However, one study did find the number of pacing runs to be associated with an increased risk of systemic inflammatory response syndrome following TAVR,[35] and systemic inflammatory response syndrome may be a risk factor for AKI following TAVR.

Contrast-Induced AKI Precautions

Most studies have not found volume of IV contrast used during TAVR to be a predictor of AKI.[13,16–18,20,26] One large study did find a relationship between contrast media dose increment and higher prevalence of AKI following TAVR.[36] They demonstrated that volume of contrast media × serum creatinine/body weight greater than 3.7 or volume of contrast media/creatinine clearance greater than 2.7 predicted AKI following TAVR. The lack of relationship between contrast volume and AKI seen in most studies likely reflects the awareness of contrast-induced AKI in this population during coronary angiography and coronary intervention with subsequent minimization of contrast use during TAVR. General precautions to prevent contrast-induced AKI, such as preprocedure and postprocedure hydration, are recommended for patients undergoing TAVR.

SUMMARY

CKD increases the risk of TAVR in the high-risk symptomatic patients that are typically referred for this procedure. In the preprocedural planning, minimizing contrast dose is critical for preventing further renal compromise before TAVR. Biplane angiography, computed tomography with intra-arterial contrast injection, use of three-dimensional TEE or CMR for annular measurement, and proper hydration before contrast administration can help to ameliorate the risk of AKI following TAVR. Minimizing contrast during the procedure and preventing hemodynamic perturbations in the operative and perioperative period are of paramount importance in decreasing the risk of AKI following TAVR. Ultimate success of TAVR depends on careful attention to detail and expeditious management of complications.[37]

REFERENCES

1. Chertow GM, Burdick E, Honour M, et al. Acute kidney injury, mortality, length of stay, and costs in hospitalized patients. J Am Soc Nephrol 2005;16: 3365–70.
2. Brennan JM, Edwards FH, Yue Z, et al. Long-term survival after aortic valve replacement among high-risk elderly patients in the United States. Insights from the Society of Thoracic Surgeons adult cardiac surgery database, 1991 to 2007. Circulation 2012; 126:1621–9.
3. Greason KL, Englberger L, Suri RM, et al. Safety of same-day coronary angiography in patients undergoing elective aortic valve replacement. Ann Thorac Surg 2011;91:1791–6.
4. Smith CR, Leon MB, Mack MJ, et al. Transcatheter versus surgical aortic-valve replacement in high-risk patients. N Engl J Med 2011;364:2187–98.
5. Smith CR, Leon MB, Mack MJ, et al. Transcatheter aortic-valve replacement for aortic stenosis in patients who cannot undergo surgery. N Engl J Med 2010;363:1597–607.
6. Cribier A, Eltchaninoff H, Bash A, et al. Percutaneous transcatheter implantation of an aortic valve prosthesis for calcific aortic stenosis: first human case description. Circulation 2002;106:3006–8.
7. Leon MB, Piazza N, Nikolsky E, et al. Standardized endpoint definitions for transcatheter aortic valve implantation clinical trials: a consensus report from the Valve Academic Research Consortium. J Am Coll Cardiol 2011;57:253–69.
8. Genereux P, Kodali SK, Green P, et al. Incidence and effect of acute kidney injury after transcatheter aortic valve replacement using the New Valve Academic Research Consortium Criteria. Am J Cardiol 2013;111:100–5.
9. Takagi H, Niwa M, Mizuno Y, et al. Incidence, predictors, and prognosis of acute kidney injury after transcatheter aortic valve implantation: a summary of contemporary studies using Valve Academic Research Consortium definitions. Int J Cardiol 2013; 168(2):1631–5.
10. Kappetein AP, Head SJ, Genereax P, et al. Updated standardized endpoint definitions for transcatheter aortic valve implantation: the Valve Academic Research Consortium-2 consensus document. J Thorac Cardiovasc Surg 2012;145:6–23.
11. Mehta RL, Kellum JA, Shah SV, et al. Acute Kidney Injury Network: report of an initiative to improve outcomes in acute kidney injury. Crit Care 2007; 11:R31.
12. Konigstein M, Ben-Assa E, Abramowitz Y, et al. Usefulness of Updated Valve Academic Research Consortium-2 criteria for acute kidney injury following transcatheter aortic valve implantation. Am J Cardiol 2013;112:1807–11.
13. Elhmidi Y, Bleiziffer S, Piazza N, et al. Incidence and predictors of acute kidney injury in patients undergoing transcatheter aortic valve implantation. Am Heart J 2011;161:735–9.
14. Khawaja MZ, Thomas M, Joshi A, et al. The effects of VARC-defined acute kidney injury after transcatheter aortic valve implantation (TAVI) using the Edwards bioprosthesis. EuroIntervention 2012;5:563–70.
15. Kong WY, Yong G, Irish A. Incidence, risk factors and prognosis of acute kidney injury after transcatheter aortic valve implantation. Nephrology (Carlton) 2012;17:445–51.
16. Aregger F, Wenaweser P, Hellige GJ, et al. Risk of acute kidney injury in patients with severe aortic valve stenosis undergoing transcatheter valve replacement. Nephrol Dial Transplant 2009;24: 2175–9.
17. Bagur R, Webb JG, Nietlispach F, et al. Acute kidney injury following transcatheter aortic valve implantation: predictive factors, prognostic value, and comparison with surgical aortic valve replacement. Eur Heart J 2010;31:865–74.
18. Barbash IM, Ben-Dor I, Dvir D, et al. Incidence and predictors of acute kidney injury after transcatheter aortic valve replacement. Am Heart J 2012;163: 1031–6.
19. Saia F, Ciuca C, Taglieri N, et al. Acute kidney injury following transcatheter aortic valve implantation: incidence, predictors and clinical outcome. Int J Cardiol 2013;168:1034–40.

20. Nuis JM, Van Mieghem NM, Tzikas A, et al. Frequency, determinants, and prognostic effects of acute kidney injury and red blood cell transfusion in patients undergoing transcatheter aortic valve implantation. Catheter Cardiovasc Interv 2011;77:881–9.

21. Nuis R, Rodes-Cabau J, Sinning J, et al. Blood transfusion and the risk of acute kidney injury after transcatheter aortic valve implantation. Circ Cardiovasc Interv 2012;5:680–8.

22. Buchanan GL, Chieffo A, Montorfano M, et al. The role of sex on VARC outcomes following transcatheter aortic valve implantation with both Edwards SAPIEN™ and Medtronic CoreValve ReValving System® devices: the Milan registry. EuroIntervention 2011;7(5):556–63.

23. Koch CG, Li L, Duncan AI, et al. Morbidity and mortality risk associated with red blood cell and blood-component transfusion in isolated coronary artery bypass grafting. Crit Care Med 2006;34:1608–16.

24. Murphy GJ, Reeves BC, Rogers CA, et al. Increased mortality, postoperative morbidity, and cost after red blood cell transfusion in patients having cardiac surgery. Circulation 2007;116:2544–52.

25. Alassar A, Roy D, Abdulkareem N, et al. Acute kidney injury after transcatheter aortic valve implantation: incidence, risk factors, and prognostic effects. Innovations 2012;7:389–93.

26. Sinning J, Ghanem A, Steinhauser H, et al. Renal function as predictor of mortality in patients after percutaneous transcatheter aortic valve implantation. JACC Cardiovasc Interv 2010;3(11):1141–9.

27. Dasta JF, Kane-Gill SL, Durtschi AJ, et al. Costs and outcomes of acute kidney injury (AKI) following cardiac surgery. Nephrol Dial Transplant 2008;23:1970–4.

28. Brandt MM, Falvo AJ, Rubinfeld IS, et al. Renal dysfunction in trauma: even a little costs a lot. J Trauma 2007;62:1362–4.

29. Kapadia SR, Schoenhagen P, Stewart W, et al. Imaging for transcatheter valve procedures. Curr Probl Cardiol 2010;35:228–76.

30. Bloomfield GS, Gillam LD, Hahn RT, et al. A practical guide to multimodality imaging of transcatheter aortic valve replacement. JACC Cardiovasc Imaging 2012;5(4):441–55.

31. Ng AC, Delgado V, van der Kley F. Comparison of aortic root dimensions and geometries before and after transcatheter aortic valve implantation by 2- and 3-dimensional transesophageal echocardiography and multislice computed tomography. Circ Cardiovasc Imaging 2010;3(1):94–102.

32. Bagur R, Rodes-Cabau J, Doyle D, et al. Usefulness of TEE as the primary imaging technique to guide transcatheter transapical aortic valve implantation. JACC Cardiovasc Imaging 2011;4(2):115–24.

33. Svensson LG, Kapadia SR, Rodriguez L, et al. Percutaneous aortic valves and imaging. JACC Cardiovasc Imaging 2011;4(2):125–7.

34. Gurvitch R, Wood DA, Tay EL. Transcatheter aortic valve implantation: durability of clinical and hemodynamic outcomes beyond 3 years in a large patient cohort. Circulation 2010;122(13):1319–27.

35. Sinning J, Scheer A, Adenauer V, et al. Systemic inflammatory response syndrome predicts increased mortality in patients after transcatheter aortic valve implantation. Eur Heart J 2012;33(12):1459–68.

36. Yamamoto M, Hayashida K, Mouillet G, et al. Renal function-based contrast dosing predicts acute kidney injury following transcatheter aortic valve implantation. JACC Cardiovasc Interv 2013;6:479–86.

37. Kapadia SR, Svensson LG, Roselli E, et al. Single center TAVR experience with a focus on the prevention and management of catastrophic complications. Catheter Cardiovasc Interv 2014;1–9. [Epub ahead of print].

Index

Note: Page numbers of article titles are in **boldface** type.

A

Ablation therapy, for atrial fibrillation, 321
N-Acetyl-β-D-glucosaminidase, as biomarker, 360–361, 384, 387
N-Acetylcysteine, for CIN prevention, 410–414, 433
ACT (Acetylcysteine for Contrast Nephropathy) trial, 410, 414, 433
ACTIVE trial, 352
Acute coronary syndrome, diagnosis of, 319
Acute kidney injury. *See* Contrast-induced acute kidney injury.
Acute Kidney Injury Network, 450
Acute Kidney Injury Network criteria, for prediction complications, 369–370
A-HEFT study, 325
Airway compromise, in contrast media hypersensitivity, 344–345
Allergic-like (anaphylactoid) reactions, to contrast media, 341–346
Alpha GST, as biomarker, 360–361
American College of Cardiology Foundation/Society for Cardiovascular Angiography and Interventions guidelines, for CIN prevention, 430–431, 433
Amiodarone, for atrial fibrillation, 321
Anaphylactoid reactions, to contrast media, 341–346
Anemia, in heart failure, 324
Angioedema, in contrast media hypersensitivity, 343
Angiotensin, in CI-AKI, 365
Angiotensin receptor blockers, for heart failure, 323
Angiotensin-converting enzyme inhibitors, nephrotoxicity of, 323–324, 433–434
Anticoagulation, for atrial fibrillation, 322
Antihypertensive drugs, for coronary artery disease, 320
Antioxidant mechanisms, fluid administration effects on, 395
Antiplatelet agents, for coronary artery disease, 319–320
Aortic interventions, renal complications in, 445–446
Aortic valve replacement, transcatheter, renal complications in, **449–454**
Apixaban, for atrial fibrillation, 322
Apoptosis, in CI-AKI, 364
ARMYDA-CIN (Atorvastatin for Reduction of Myocardial Damage during Angioplasty-contrast-Induced Nephropathy) trial, 409
Arrhythmias, from contrast media, 341
Ascorbic acid, for CIN prevention, 414–415

Aspiration system, for contrast media removal, 424–425
Aspirin, for coronary artery disease, 319–320
Atheroembolization, of renal artery, 445
Atherosclerosis
  coronary, 318–321
  peripheral, 451
Atorvastatin, for CI-AKI prevention, 406–407, 409
Atorvastatin for Reduction of Myocardial Damage during Angioplasty-contrast-Induced Nephropathy (ARMYDA-CIN) trial, 409
Atrial fibrillation, chronic kidney disease with, 321–322
Atropine, for contrast media hypersensitivity, 344–345
Attallah trial, of CI-AKI prevention, 407
Automated balanced hydration, 423, 425
AVERT contrast injection device, 422

B

Bader trial, of fluid administration methods, 397–398
Balloon(s), for contrast media removal, 424–425
Bartholomew risk score, 371, 373
Benephit catheter, 426
Beta blockers
  for atrial fibrillation, 321
  for contrast media hypersensitivity, 344
  for coronary artery disease, 320
  for heart failure, 323–324
Bicarbonate, 397, 402, 432–434, 443–444
Bicarbonate or Saline Study (BOSS), 402
Biomarkers, for CI-AKI and CIN, 359–361, **379–391**
  clinical relevance of, 387–388
  clinical studies of, 385–387
  examples of, 381–385
  history of, 380–381
  ideal qualities of, 379
BioPorto assay, for neutrophil gelatinase-associated lipocalin, 384–385
Bisoprolol, for atrial fibrillation, 321
Bleeding, in TAVR, 451
Blood transfusions, in TAVR, 451
Blue Cross Blue Shield of Michigan Cardiovascular Consortium registry, 432
BMC1 risk model, 430–431
BOSS (Bicarbonate or Saline Study), 402
Bouzas-Mosquera trial, of CI-AKI prevention, 407

Moving?

Make sure your subscription moves with you!

To notify us of your new address, find your **Clinics Account Number** (located on your mailing label above your name), and contact customer service at:

Email: journalscustomerservice-usa@elsevier.com

800-654-2452 (subscribers in the U.S. & Canada)
314-447-8871 (subscribers outside of the U.S. & Canada)

Fax number: 314-447-8029

Elsevier Health Sciences Division
Subscription Customer Service
3251 Riverport Lane
Maryland Heights, MO 63043

*To ensure uninterrupted delivery of your subscription, please notify us at least 4 weeks in advance of move.

Printed and bound by CPI Group (UK) Ltd, Croydon, CR0 4YY

03/10/2024

01040379-0011